Navigating Life with Multiple Sclerosis

David Spencer, MD, FAAN

Editor, *Brain & Life*® Books Series
Professor of Neurology
Oregon Health and Science University
Portland, OR

Other Titles in the *Brain & Life*® Books Series

Navigating Life with a Brain Tumor
Lynne P. Taylor, MD, FAAN; Alyx B. Porter Umphrey, MD; and
Diane Richard

Navigating the Complexities of Stroke
Louis R. Caplan, MD, FAAN

Navigating Life with Epilepsy
David C. Spencer, MD, FAAN

Navigating Life with Amyotrophic Lateral Sclerosis
Mark B. Bromberg, MD, PhD, FAAN; and Diane Banks Bromberg, JD

Navigating Life with Migraine and Other Headaches
William B. Young, MD, FAAN, FANA, FAHS; and Stephen D. Silberstein,
MD, FAHS, FAAN, FACP

Navigating Life with Chronic Pain
Robert A. Lavin, MD, MS; Sara Clayton, PhD; and Lindsay Zilliox, MD

Navigating Life with Parkinson's Disease, Second Edition
Sotirios A. Parashos, MD; and Rose Wichmann, PT

Navigating Life with Dementia
James M. Noble, MD, MS, CPH, FAAN

Navigating the Challenges of Concussion
Michael S. Jaffee, MD, FAAN, FANA; Donna K. Broshek, PhD, ABPP-CN;
and Adrian M. Svingos, PhD

Navigating Life with Restless Legs Syndrome
Andrew R. Spector, MD

Navigating Life with Multiple Sclerosis

SECOND EDITION

Kathleen Costello, MS, CRNP, MSCN
Chief Operating Officer, Can Do Multiple Sclerosis

Rosalind Kalb, PhD, CHC
Senior Programs Consultant, Can Do Multiple Sclerosis

Barbara S. Giesser, MD, FAAN, FANA
Professor Emeritus of Clinical Neurology, University of California, Los Angeles

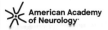 American Academy of Neurology

OXFORD
UNIVERSITY PRESS

OXFORD
UNIVERSITY PRESS

Oxford University Press is a department of the University of Oxford. It furthers the University's objective of excellence in research, scholarship, and education by publishing worldwide. Oxford is a registered trade mark of Oxford University Press in the UK and certain other countries.

Published in the United States of America by Oxford University Press
198 Madison Avenue, New York, NY 10016, United States of America.

© American Academy of Neurology 2025

CIP data is on file at the Library of Congress

This material is not intended to be, and should not be considered, a substitute for medical or other professional advice. Treatment for the conditions described in this material is highly dependent on the individual circumstances. And, while this material is designed to offer accurate information with respect to the subject matter covered and to be current as of the time it was written, research and knowledge about medical and health issues is constantly evolving and dose schedules for medications are being revised continually, with new side effects recognized and accounted for regularly. Readers must therefore always check the product information and clinical procedures with the most up-to-date published product information and data sheets provided by the manufacturers and the most recent codes of conduct and safety regulation. The publisher and the authors make no representations or warranties to readers, express or implied, as to the accuracy or completeness of this material. Without limiting the foregoing, the publisher and the authors make no representations or warranties as to the accuracy or efficacy of the drug dosages mentioned in the material. The authors and the publisher do not accept, and expressly disclaim, any responsibility for any liability, loss or risk that may be claimed or incurred as a consequence of the use and/or application of any of the contents of this material.

ISBN 978-0-19-774869-5

DOI: 10.1093/oso/9780197748695.001.0001

Printed by Sheridan Books, Inc., United States of America

We dedicate Navigating Life with Multiple Sclerosis to the many people with MS and their care partners who have trusted us to be a part of their care. Your courage, determination, and resilience have been a source of inspiration to us. To those living with MS, we honor your strength and perseverance in facing many daily challenges of MS. To care partners, we thank you for the support and care you have provided. Thank you for allowing us to share in your experiences and partner with you in your MS journey.

CONTENTS

Section 3: Health and Wellness

ABOUT THE *BRAIN & LIFE*®
BOOKS SERIES

What was the first thing you thought when you learned you or a family member had a neurologic disease? Perhaps you were confused, uncertain, afraid, or maybe even in denial. A common thread is often the realization that life has changed and may continue to change, but also uncertainty about exactly what that means or what to expect. And yet, neurologic diseases themselves inevitably change—sometimes quickly, in a matter of seconds or minutes, and sometimes gradually over months or even years.

With any new diagnosis—especially one that is potentially life-changing—you may not be prepared to take in and process large amounts of new information on the spot. And even under the best circumstances, each condition comes with the need to learn a new language and understand the necessary tests, underlying causes, and right treatments. It may be difficult to wrap your arms around a great deal of information in what are often time-limited appointments with your neurologist. Understanding your new diagnosis and how to manage it is a gradual process, and you will inevitably have questions with the passage of time and reflection. Learning about your condition can help you understand what the most useful and accurate information is to share with your neurology team, allowing you to fully participate in treatment decisions.

But facts and information are only part of the picture. You may have questions about how to manage your day-to-day life with a neurologic disease: whether in terms of your career, your home, your relationships, or, in some instances, long-term planning and care. We designed the *Brain & Life* Books series to help you address some of the fears, concerns, and difficult emotions you may feel, such as grief and worry, by harnessing the power of accurate and timely information to help guide you and your family through the change brought about by a neurologic diagnosis. The books share stories of others who have traveled down paths like the one you are on to reinforce the fact that you are not alone.

We selected the authors of the series carefully with these goals in mind. First and foremost, all authors are respected experts in their field, and the information in the *Brain & Life* Books series is accurate, up-to-date, and written to be understandable to someone with no medical background. Experts from the leading professional neurology organization in the world—the American Academy of Neurology—and the oldest and largest university press in the world—Oxford University Press—carefully review each book to ensure the highest quality. But we also chose our authors because of their experience and ability to connect with patients and their families. The experiences and feelings you are having now have been dealt with and managed successfully by our authors and their patients. Our authors will share with you best practices, stories, and pearls of advice that will leave you with a feeling that your diagnosis is manageable—you can do this. We have highlighted all key terms that you and your family should know when first used, and we have included them in a comprehensive glossary at the back of the book.

The *Brain & Life* Books series was written with you in mind, whether you have been diagnosed yourself or are a family member, caregiver, or friend of someone who has been, as a resource for successfully navigating life with a neurologic disease.

David Spencer, MD, FAAN
Editor, *Brain & Life*® Books Series
Professor of Neurology
Oregon Health and Science University
Portland, OR

PREFACE: NAVIGATING LIFE WITH MS 2ND EDITION

In the 10 years that have passed since the first edition of Navigating Life with MS was published, we have seen major advancements in the ability to diagnose & treat MS, an increased focus on overall health and wellness as a component of comprehensive MS care, and a deeper understanding of the impact of a chronic, unpredictable illness on the entire family. Our ongoing effort is to provide you with the information and resources you need to live optimally with MS, whether you are dealing with a new diagnosis, adjusting to changes caused by the disease, or are learning together with your care partner(s) (spouse, partner, parent, adult child, or friend) how to communicate effectively and support one another. This information also will help you to become a more active and informed participant in your healthcare provider's treatment decisions.

We have updated all of the existing chapters in the book with the latest information and added new ones that address emotional and cognitive challenges, changes in sexual function, and relationships and communication – with one another and with members of your healthcare team – and planning for unpredictability. Our updated information about the role of wellness in MS management provides current recommendations about diet and exercise, as well as information about ways to prevent or manage other health conditions that can impact MS progression. Living well with MS requires multi-disciplinary teamwork, with you at the center. We sincerely hope that this 2nd edition helps you navigate your life with MS.

Kathy Costello, Barbara Giesser and Roz Kalb

FOREWORD: NAVIGATING LIFE WITH MS 2ND EDITION

Living with multiple sclerosis (MS) is a journey marked by challenges, uncertainties, and moments of profound resilience. As someone who has not only navigated this journey personally but also dedicated my professional life to understanding and treating this complex condition, I am deeply moved by the effort the authors devoted to making this invaluable resource. The blend of clear information, education, and practical advice resonates deeply with my experiences as both a patient and a healthcare provider, and makes it an essential tool for navigating life with MS.

My own MS diagnosis came with a flood of questions, fears, and a pressing need for reliable information. This guide would have been such a comfort during that time! The authors provide essential knowledge with compassion and clarity and provide a roadmap for managing MS throughout one's life. MS is not a one-size-fits-all condition but a deeply personal experience that is ever changing. From fatigue and mobility issues to sensory symptoms and cognitive changes, each chapter delves into the nuances of living with MS. These sections do more than just provide information; they offer resources, actionable strategies, and insights that can significantly improve quality of life no matter what MS throws our way. The emphasis on care partners is also testament to the fact that MS is not just an individual experience but a collective one. It offers guidance and support for those who stand by our side, ensuring they are equipped to navigate this path with us. As a lifelong disease, MS remains a constant presence as we age. Our needs and priorities inevitably change as our families, careers, and interests evolve. I love that this book can be a valuable resource at every stage of our lives with MS. Whether you are newly diagnosed or have lived with MS for decades, it offers relevant and practical advice. Each time you revisit its pages, you will discover new insights and strategies that reflect your current experiences and needs, making it a timeless companion for living well with MS.

As someone who sees MS from both sides of the desk, I believe this book is an indispensable guide. It bridges the gap between medical knowledge and real-life application that people affected by MS can use as a resource throughout their lives. This book not only informs but also empowers, offering hope and practical solutions for living well with MS. It is more than just a book; it is a companion for anyone living with MS, offering insights, support, and a sense of community.

With heartfelt appreciation,
Stephanie Buxhoeveden, PhD, MSN, FNP-BC, MSCN

Overview of
Multiple Sclerosis

CHAPTER 1

What Is Multiple Sclerosis?

In this chapter, you will learn:

- What the term "multiple sclerosis" means
- Who is likely to get multiple sclerosis
- What causes multiple sclerosis
- What are the risk factors for developing multiple sclerosis
- What are the courses that multiple sclerosis can take over time

Because you are reading this book, it is likely that you, a family member, or someone else significant to you has been diagnosed with **multiple sclerosis (MS)**. Perhaps you have lived with MS for years but continue to search for new information about your condition and ways to manage it.

No matter where you are on your journey with MS, this book is intended to guide you through the questions you may have and the decisions you may need to make. Our goal is to give you the answers you need and lead you to resources that will help you along the way.

If you are like many people with MS, it may have taken months or even years for you to get this diagnosis. Because the symptoms of the disease can come and go unpredictably, people often live with them for years—and may receive several different diagnoses—before their condition is finally identified.

So What Is Multiple Sclerosis, Anyway?

Multiple sclerosis is a chronic disease that affects the body's **central nervous system (CNS)**, which includes the brain, **spinal cord**, and **optic nerves** (Figure 1.1). It is an **autoimmune disease**, which means

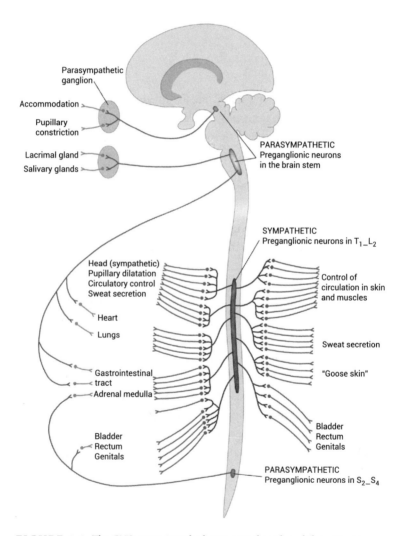

FIGURE 1.1 The CNS comprises the brain, spinal cord, and the optic nerve.

that the body's **immune system** mistakenly attacks and damages healthy **nerves** and other cells in the CNS. This damage interrupts transmission of messages between nerves in the CNS and the rest of the body, which can produce many different symptoms, including **multiple sclerosis (MS) fatigue, numbness, spasticity,** weakness, vision changes, loss of balance, mood changes, and problems with thinking and memory, among others.

Multiple sclerosis was first described formally in 1868 by the French **neurologist** Jean-Martin Charcot, a clinical and scientific pioneer known as the founder of modern **neurology**. Integrating his clinical and anatomic observations with earlier reports from other 19th-century neurologists, he named the condition *la sclérose en plaques disséminées* (disseminated **sclerosis**). Areas of scarring (sclerosis) caused by nerve damage in the CNS are technically known as **plaques** but are more commonly referred to as **lesions**. These lesions can be visualized on **magnetic resonance imaging (MRI)**.

What Happens in Multiple Sclerosis?

The basic problem in MS is abnormal function of the immune system. Normally, the immune system, which is made up of different types of cells (primarily white blood cells) and immune proteins, protects a person's body or "self" from "foreign" and potentially harmful things in the outside environment, such as bacteria and viruses. In an autoimmune disease such as MS, the immune system becomes confused and mistakenly attacks a part of the "self" that it now recognizes as "foreign." There are dozens of autoimmune diseases. In some forms of diabetes, the immune system attacks the pancreas. In rheumatoid arthritis, the targets are joints. In MS, the immune system damages the nerves in the CNS.

Normally, the CNS is what is called an "immunologically privileged" site, meaning that immune cells generally do not enter the CNS in a healthy individual. But in a person with MS, they gain access to the CNS and cause damage. MS treatments, or **disease-modifying therapies (DMTs)** (see Chapter 3), work by interfering with the immune system's ability to enter the CNS and attack the nerves.

In MS, the main CNS target of the immune system is a substance called **myelin**, which forms a protective sheath around the **nerve fibers** known as **axons**—the primary transmission lines for the electrical signals (messages) within the nervous system. The axons, as well as **oligodendrocytes** (the cells that make myelin in the CNS), can also be damaged or destroyed in MS (Figure 1.2).

Lesions form where the damage has occurred. The damage to myelin and axons disrupts or stops the electrical and chemical signals transmitted from one **nerve cell** to the next. Think of it as a downed power line: When that power line is damaged or cut, it cannot transmit the signal telling your refrigerator or telephone to turn on. Similarly, if enough nerve cells are damaged in your CNS, signals that tell you to move your arm or maintain your balance can be interrupted.

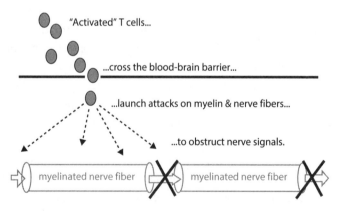

FIGURE 1.2 Cells of the immune system entering the CNS and causing inflammation and damage.

Who Gets Multiple Sclerosis?

You are probably wondering why you or your loved one got MS. Although there is not a simple answer, we know approximately how many people develop MS and which members of the population are more likely to be affected.

According to the National Multiple Sclerosis Society, approximately 1 million people in the United States today are living with MS. About 10,000 new cases are diagnosed each year—or 200 people every week. Worldwide, the disease affects an estimated 2.8 million people. Most people with MS are diagnosed between ages 15 and 50 years, and while most of those cases occur between ages 20 and 40 years, about 10% of people with MS develop symptoms before age 18 years.

Multiple sclerosis affects three times as many women as men. For reasons that are not yet entirely clear, most autoimmune diseases are more common in women. Recent research suggests that this may be a result of profound effects of **sex hormones** and **sex chromosomes** on immune function.

For years, MS has been considered more common in White people, particularly White women of northern European descent. However, data from a large Southern California study have challenged that theory. These data showed the highest prevalence of MS in Black women, followed by White women, with lower rates in Hispanic and Asian individuals.

What Causes Multiple Sclerosis?

The exact cause of MS remains unknown. However, researchers have looked at many factors that seem to be involved.

The Role of Genetics

In the general population, the risk of developing MS is about 1 in 334 people. A person who has a first-degree relative with MS, such as a parent or sibling, has about a 4% chance of developing MS. Should both parents have MS, each of their children has a 30–35% chance of developing MS. And in identical twins, if one twin has MS, there is a 30% chance that the other twin will develop MS as well.

It is important to note that while some **genetic** association exists, there is no conclusive evidence that the disease is inherited from a parent through **gene** transmission. However, several studies have identified certain genes that control the development and function of many of the immune system processes that are known to be abnormal in people with MS. Many risk genes have been identified, each making a small contribution to the overall risk of developing MS.

The Role of Climate and Vitamin D

For reasons that are not completely understood, the farther one lives from the equator, the greater the chances of developing MS. Countries such as the United States, Canada, Europe, Australia, and New Zealand have a higher risk of MS than other countries with less temperate climates. This is thought to be due, at least in part, to reduced sunlight exposure and **vitamin D** production in those areas.

Scientists have studied the impact of low vitamin D on the risk of MS. Naturally produced vitamin D, which is created by exposure to sunlight, is thought to have a beneficial effect on the immune system and thus may protect against autoimmune diseases such as MS. Given that people who move from a darker, more northern climate to a sunnier one at an early age acquire the relative risk for MS found in their new, adopted climate, it makes sense that something about vitamin D levels during a certain key period of childhood and young adulthood plays a role in developing MS. Many different studies have reported that low sunlight exposure in early childhood, and thus lower vitamin D levels during this time, appears to correlate with an increased risk of developing MS later in life.

Many researchers think that in addition to the genetic and climate factors we have already mentioned, there are several risk factors that increase a person's chances of getting MS.

Exposure to a Virus or Viruses

Viruses are thought to have a possible link to MS; however, this does not mean that MS is contagious. There are two ways in which a virus might cause nerve damage that is seen in MS:

1. A virus might attack the nervous system directly.
2. The virus can cause damage indirectly. When a virus enters the body, the immune system becomes activated to fight its invasion. If some parts of the virus are similar to some parts of the CNS, the immune system will mistakenly attack the CNS as well.

Recent **epidemiologic studies** suggest that exposure to **Epstein–Barr virus (EBV)**, the virus that causes **mononucleosis**, may be a necessary (but not sufficient) factor for developing MS. In other words, exposure to the virus must occur in order for MS to develop, but the virus alone is not enough to cause the disease to become active. Even after the acute infection is gone, EBV remains in certain immune cells and continues to stimulate an immune response. In addition, some of the proteins on the virus are similar to proteins found in myelin, which triggers the immune system to attack the myelin by mistake. Vaccines against EBV are in development, which means that in the future, many new cases of MS may be prevented.

Lifestyle Factors

Recent research findings suggest that smoking increases the risk for developing MS, including secondhand smoke and even prenatal exposure. There are also studies that have reported that people who are obese as children, adolescents, or young adults have a higher risk of developing MS. While these observations are not yet definitive, they underscore the importance of maintaining a healthy lifestyle and may hold important clues to the underlying mechanisms that produce nerve damage in MS.

What Happens in Multiple Sclerosis Over Time?

Multiple sclerosis does not have a single, predictable disease course. The nature of MS and the patterns it takes change over time and vary from person to person. The damage in the CNS caused by the immune system drives disease activity, relapses, progression, and accumulation of disability over a person's lifetime with MS.

In an effort to help the entire MS community better understand what happens in MS over time, the National Multiple Sclerosis Society and the European Committee for Treatment and Research for Multiple Sclerosis organized an international committee to define a classification of disease courses that includes **clinically isolated syndrome (CIS)**; **relapsing–remitting MS (RRMS)**; and **progressive MS**, which is further divided into **primary progressive MS (PPMS)** and **secondary progressive MS (SPMS)**. In addition to the broad classifications, additional clarification based on whether the disease is active (relapses and/or new lesions on MRI) and whether MS is progressing or not is now part of the disease course classification (Figure 1.3). Although not included in this formal classification, there is a "pre-MS" type known as **radiologically isolated syndrome (RIS)**, which is described in greater detail in Chapter 2.

Let us take a closer look at the three disease courses of MS.

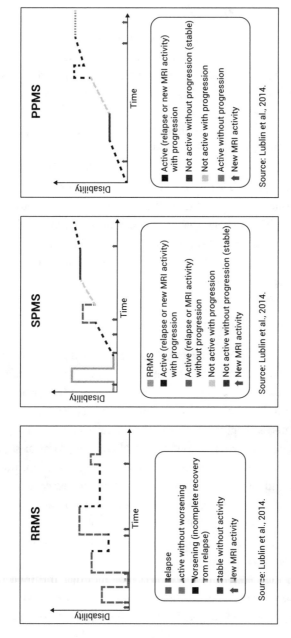

FIGURE 1.3 Relapsing–remitting MS (RRMS), secondary progressive MS (SPMS), and primary progressive MS (PPMS). Reprinted with permission of the National Multiple Sclerosis Society.

Clinically Isolated Syndrome

When someone has a first neurologic episode that is consistent with CNS inflammation, it is considered a CIS. Most, but not all, people who experience CIS will later develop more symptoms and more evidence of CNS inflammation, leading to a diagnosis of MS.

- A CIS is a clinical symptom or symptoms that arise from an abnormality in the brain, spinal cord, or optic nerve.
- It can involve one symptom, such as visual loss in one eye, or more than one symptom, such as weakness and visual symptoms that occur at the same time. While the symptoms could be highly suggestive of MS, they must be separated in space (in the CNS) and time in order to meet criteria or "rules" for an MS diagnosis. More information about how MS is diagnosed is presented in Chapter 2.

Relapsing–Remitting Multiple Sclerosis

Relapsing–remitting MS, the most common MS disease course, is characterized by clearly defined attacks of neurologic symptoms (**relapses, exacerbations**, attacks, or flares), followed by periods with partial or complete recovery (**remissions**). Between 85% and 90% of individuals newly diagnosed with MS have a relapsing–remitting disease course. A **relapse** refers to new neurologic symptoms or significant worsening of existing neurologic symptoms that last a minimum of 24 hours and cannot be explained by any other cause, such as an infection, heat, humidity, or exertion. During these relapses, neurologic function is impaired—for example, a person may have great difficulty walking without tripping or may find it difficult to see clearly out of one eye.

Relapses generally last several weeks or months, and then they begin to resolve or disappear during a period of remission. Symptoms may go away completely or partially. After a relapse subsides, periods of time—months or years—may pass during which no new symptoms typical of a relapse occur. Recovery may or may not be 100%, and recovery is often better early in the disease. When recovery is less than 100%, it is considered incomplete, and the symptoms that remain are referred to as **residual symptoms.**

Susan was diagnosed with MS after experiencing an episode of **optic neuritis** *(inflammation of the optic [vision] nerve causing blurred or dim vision or complete loss of vision in one eye) that was followed 6 months later by numbness in both her legs.*

The optic neuritis began when Susan awoke one morning and noticed that the vision in her left eye was blurry, as though her contact lens was dirty. And when she looked around, she had an achy **sensation** *behind that eye. She saw an* **ophthalmologist** *and was found to have visual acuity or sharpness of vision of 20/200 in the left eye as well as impaired* **color vision**—*both findings being characteristic of optic neuritis.*

After about 6 weeks, the optic neuritis went away, and Susan recovered her vision almost completely. Because optic neuritis can be a common first symptom of MS, Susan's ophthalmologist referred her to a neurologist, who ordered an MRI scan of her brain. The MRI showed evidence of lesions in the brain that were compatible with MS.

In addition, some of the lesions in the brain were inflamed, and some were not. Because of these MRI findings, updated **diagnostic criteria** *allowed Susan to be diagnosed with MS even though she had experienced only one attack. (See Chapter 2.)*

Six months later, Susan woke up with a numb left foot. Over the next 2 days, this numbness spread to both legs and up to her waist. These symptoms persisted for 4 weeks and then subsided, leaving a slight numbness in her left large toe. She has not experienced any additional symptoms since that time.

Susan's optic neuritis and episode of numbness are examples of relapses.

Progressive Multiple Sclerosis

Secondary Progressive Multiple Sclerosis

The initial course of RRMS may be followed by a course of SPMS, in which the disease worsens over time and may include periods of stability and occasional relapses (particularly early in the secondary progressive course).

Research in people who had not been treated with a DMT showed that 50–65% of those with RRMS transitioned to SPMS within about 10–15 years of the first symptom and that about 90% did so within 20 years. The number of people who transition to SPMS has been reduced by the use of DMTs, which first became available in 1993 (see Chapter 3). To most of us, the word "progression," when linked to a disease, sounds ominous, and many people with MS may worry that life in a wheelchair lies ahead. However, that is not always how things end up. In fact, even though some people with RRMS will move on to a secondary progressive disease course, far fewer will ultimately need a wheelchair.

Jane was diagnosed with MS when she was 31 years old. During the next 10 years, she experienced four relapses, including a band of numbness around her waist, weakness of her right arm and leg, optic neuritis in her left eye, and clumsiness of her left arm and hand. Each of these relapses lasted several weeks and then remitted over several more weeks. Jane had incomplete recovery from two of the relapses and continued to experience mild weakness in her right arm and leg and occasional numbness around her waist.

Following her last relapse, Jane noticed that over the next 2 years, her walking endurance declined, and she slowly developed more weakness in her right arm and her legs, to the point that she now sometimes trips over her right foot when walking. She also finds that she can no longer hold objects with just her right hand. As time has passed, she has begun to need to use a cane when walking farther than two blocks.

Jane's MS can now be described as secondary progressive. She had clear relapses early in the disease, but after 10 years, she began to have a decline in function without experiencing another obvious relapse.

Primary Progressive Multiple Sclerosis

Primary progressive MS is a disease course marked by a decline in neurologic function from the start, with very few relapses or remissions. Approximately 10% of people with MS are diagnosed with PPMS. The disease course may plateau or even temporarily improve at times, but the symptoms generally do not go away completely.

Unlike the other types of MS, PPMS appears to affect men just as often as women. The initial onset of PPMS also differs somewhat from other forms of the disease; it tends to be diagnosed more often after age 40 years, about 10 years later than RRMS.

PPMS almost always affects the spinal cord, which tends to produce problems with walking and bladder, bowel, and sexual function. Individuals with this type of MS often experience difficulties over time with their ability to walk. Someone diagnosed with PPMS may need the assistance of a cane or crutch when walking earlier in the disease course than someone with RRMS.

Steve, who is in his mid-40s, began to experience problems during his daily 5-mile run. His legs became unnaturally stiff and tired, and he needed to shorten his run to 3 miles. He also noticed that his legs tingled when he jogged. The symptoms seemed to go away about 4 hours after he finished a run, only to return the next time he went out. Over a period of 18 months, the tingling and stiffness increased. But he did not seek medical help until his wife, after noticing that his manner of walking seemed to be growing unsteady, persuaded him to see his primary care physician. The doctor watched Steve walk and then tested his strength and **reflexes.** *She asked if he had ever experienced double vision, vision loss, muscle weakness, or other neurologically related problems. He was unable to recall having had any such difficulties. The doctor referred Steve to a neurologist, who performed an MRI that revealed the kinds of lesions in both the brain and spinal cord that MS produces.*

Seeing the lesions that are typical of MS, the neurologist also performed a lumbar puncture ("spinal tap") and numerous blood tests to exclude other diseases. After evaluating the various test data, the neurologist told Steve that he had PPMS, based on the fact that there had been no definitive relapsing–remitting pattern, Steve's neurologic symptoms had worsened relatively slowly from the time he had first seen clues of a problem during his daily run, the MRI showed evidence of lesions in the brain and spinal cord, and the spinal fluid showed evidence of abnormalities typically seen in MS.

What Type of Multiple Sclerosis Do I Have?

The course of the disease is not always simple to define. This is particularly true when trying to distinguish between RRMS and SPMS. Both incomplete relapse recovery and disease progression can lead to the accumulation of disability. The course of the disease often becomes clearer with the passage of time.

Each of the disease course classifications is based on clinical findings—meaning how an individual is functioning, and how symptoms appear, improve, or worsen over time. More is learned every year about the **pathology** of MS—meaning what and how damage occurs within the CNS. Early MS is characterized by **inflammation** that disrupts nerve transmission and often causes episodes of symptoms or relapses. Later MS is characterized by less inflammation and fewer relapses, but it is often associated with disease **progression**. When symptoms from a relapse do not resolve completely, there can be **worsening** of function and potential disability. This has been termed **relapse-associated worsening (RAW)**. In addition to worsening from a relapse, continued underlying disease activity within the CNS that causes progression independent of relapses (PIRA) can also cause loss of function and disability. In 2022, the term **smoldering MS** was introduced to describe the underlying disease activity occurring in the CNS. Researchers have identified additional immune system cells that are associated with smoldering MS, and these may be future targets for MS treatments focusing on progression.

People newly diagnosed with MS often summon up mental pictures of the disease based on prior knowledge and past impressions. The image of a family member, friend, acquaintance, or public figure with MS will likely come to mind first. Often, these initial images prompt fear. The first question most people with a new diagnosis of MS ask their neurologists is, "When will I be in a wheelchair?" People worry whether they will be able to continue working, raising their families, and participating in all the other activities that make up their lives.

While it is true that MS is a chronic and currently incurable disease—meaning that, once diagnosed, it will remain with you for the rest of your life—it is neither a death sentence nor a one-way ticket to a wheelchair. With current DMTs and attention to overall wellness, most people with MS lead productive and satisfying lives—having children, pursuing careers, and enjoying sports and hobbies.

Summary

Multiple sclerosis is a complex disease of the CNS that is caused by abnormal function of the immune system. Much has been learned about MS since it was first described in a formal scientific fashion in 1868. However, important questions such as what causes MS have not been completely answered. Although MS is a chronic condition that a person will live with for the rest of their life, it is not generally fatal, and it does not inevitably cause significant **disability**. Due to effective MS DMTs that can limit new relapses and slow nerve damage, more effective symptom management, and careful attention to their overall health, most people with MS lead full and productive lives.

It is never too early or too late to build your support network of knowledgeable MS experts, credible resources (see Appendix 2), and the MS community.

CHAPTER 2

Diagnosing Multiple Sclerosis

In this chapter, you will learn:

- What the "rules" are for making a diagnosis of multiple sclerosis
- Why your health care provider has recommended certain tests, examinations, and procedures

You may have already been diagnosed with multiple sclerosis (MS), or you may currently be involved in the diagnostic process. In either case, it may seem confusing and uncertain. Let's start with some basic information about the process for diagnosing MS.

Why Diagnosing Multiple Sclerosis Can Be Challenging

First, there is no one test that can determine whether a person has MS. Your **MS care provider** (most often a neurologist, **physician assistant [PA]**, and/or **nurse practitioner [NP]**) uses your medical history, a comprehensive **neurologic exam**, and a variety of tests to help make the diagnosis.

Second, many medical conditions can cause symptoms similar to those seen in MS. This means that the MS care provider needs to rule out every other possible explanation of a person's symptoms before making the MS diagnosis, including **neuromyelitis optica spectrum disorder (NMOSD)**, **myelin oligodendrocyte glycoprotein** antibody-associated disease (MOGAD), other inflammatory conditions, and some infections.

Why Making the Diagnosis of Multiple Sclerosis as Soon as Possible Is Important

The symptoms of MS (see Chapters 4–9) are just the tip of the iceberg. The true extent of the disease includes not only these symptoms but also the inflammatory disease process that is at work within your central nervous system, damaging the myelin sheath around the nerve fibers, the nerve fibers themselves, and the cells that make the myelin. (For more information about the MS disease process, refer to Chapter 1.) By the time the first symptoms appear, this disease process has been ongoing for some time. Given the importance of early diagnosis and treatment of MS, researchers are looking for ways to make an accurate diagnosis as quickly as possible. An incorrect MS diagnosis may lead to unnecessary treatment of the wrong health issue.

Extensive research has shown that people with MS who start treatment with a disease-modifying therapy (DMT) early will tend to have better overall outcomes. The goal of these treatments is to reduce the number of relapses (also called attacks, flares, or exacerbations), slow the disease process, and reduce the risk of increasing disability (see Chapter 3).

Let's look at the diagnostic process in more detail.

The "Rules" or Diagnostic Criteria for Making the Multiple Sclerosis Diagnosis

The disease is called "multiple sclerosis" for good reason, as seen in the following "rules" for making the MS diagnosis:

1. There must be objective evidence that damage has occurred in more than one location in the central nervous system (CNS: brain, spinal cord, and optic nerves) (this is referred to as "**separation in space**"). The objective evidence might include abnormal findings on a neurologic examination and/or evidence of neurologic damage on magnetic resonance imaging (MRI) scans of the CNS that is consistent with MS. MS cannot be diagnosed on the basis of symptoms alone.

2. There must also be evidence that this damage occurred at different times (known as "**separation in time**"). For example, a person who had a brief episode of leg numbness a year ago may, this year, have an episode of vision loss in one eye.

3. The diagnosis can only be made when other possible explanations for the symptoms and test findings have been excluded.

The Tools a Provider Uses to Make the Diagnosis

A complex disease such as MS requires a full set of diagnostic tools as well as careful attention to the criteria for making the diagnosis.

It's been said that a provider's most important diagnostic tool is the personal medical history that a patient brings to the appointment. The first thing a provider will do when evaluating you for possible MS or any other diagnosis is to take a detailed history of symptoms you currently have and those you have experienced in the past. Common questions may include the following:

- When did the symptoms begin?
- Have you ever had them before?
- Do the symptoms interfere with your usual activities?
- What have you done to reduce the symptoms?
- Have your interventions helped?
- Have you had any recent infections?
- Have you been diagnosed with any other illnesses recently?

- Do you have any allergies—to medications, foods, or something in the environment (grass, trees, cats, etc.)?
- What medications, vitamins, or other dietary supplements do you take, and why?
- Have you ever had any other symptoms that might be characteristic of a CNS problem?
- Have any family members had similar symptoms or been diagnosed with MS or any other neurologic or autoimmune diseases such as rheumatoid arthritis or lupus?

They will also ask about your lifestyle and habits, including

- diet;
- exercise; and
- use of tobacco, alcohol, or other recreational substances.

When considering your answers to all of these questions, the provider will also take into account what is known about who typically develops MS (see Chapter 1). While young children and older adults can be diagnosed with MS, an 80-year-old man with new neurologic symptoms is more likely to have something other than MS. This knowledge can be helpful when considering a possible diagnosis.

After collecting your medical history, the provider will conduct a neurological examination (exam), which is a systematic assessment of your neurological function. The exam will assess your vision, speech, face and neck mobility, swallowing, strength, balance, walking, and sensation. During the neurologic exam, the provider is looking for clues that may point either toward or away from a diagnosis of MS. The diagnosis of MS cannot be made until other possible explanations for your neurologic symptoms can be ruled out.

Let's look at the specifics of the neurological exam.

One of the first areas that the provider will check is the function of the **cranial nerves**. These are specialized nerves that control mobility and sensation in the head, face, and neck. They allow us to see and hear clearly; feel sensation on our face; and move our eyes, head, neck, mouth, tongue, and shoulders. The provider will likely test your visual acuity with an eye chart and use an instrument called an **ophthalmoscope** to evaluate the appearance of the back of your eye or **fundus**. This examination provides valuable information about the optic nerves that carry visual information to the vision center of the brain and are often affected by MS.

The provider will also test your arm and leg mobility, strength, coordination, and your ability to walk. Strength is tested by your ability to resist the provider while they move your extremities. Also, when moving your limbs, the provider can tell if there is excess stiffness present, known as spasticity.

The provider will gently tap certain places on your arms and legs with a rubber hammer to test your **deep tendon reflexes**, which are typically overactive in people with MS. In addition to overactive reflexes, the provider is checking for abnormal reflexes, such as the **Babinski sign**, in which the big toe turns upward and the other toes fan out when the provider strokes the underside of the foot. Walking can be assessed by observing your normal walking, fast walking, distance walked, and walking heel to toe.

Pain and temperature sensitivity, response to light touch, **position sense**, **discriminative sense**, and **vibratory sense** are all different types of sensation that are typically assessed during the neurological exam. Assessing sensation is done systematically so that any change in sensation can be localized to a specific area of the nervous system.

The health care provider may also do some simple tests to assess your memory and thinking, especially if you or your family members have noticed any difficulties in these areas.

Findings from the history and the neurological exam are key to making a correct diagnosis. These findings may prompt the provider to order certain types of tests to further understand and determine the cause of the symptoms you are experiencing.

The Tests Most Often Used in Making the Multiple Sclerosis Diagnosis

Magnetic Resonance Imaging (MRI)

If your history of neurologic symptoms, together with the findings of your neurologic exam, suggests CNS damage as a cause of the symptoms, the MS care provider will likely order an MRI of your brain and the upper (**cervical**) and lower two-thirds (**thoracic**) sections of your spinal cord.

During an MRI, you must lie flat and very still on a table that slides into the narrow tube of the scanner (Figure 2.1). A brain MRI takes about 40 minutes; an MRI of the spinal cord takes about 40–60 minutes. If you are uncomfortable or anxious in enclosed spaces, you must inform your MS care provider ahead of time so that a mild sedative can be prescribed.

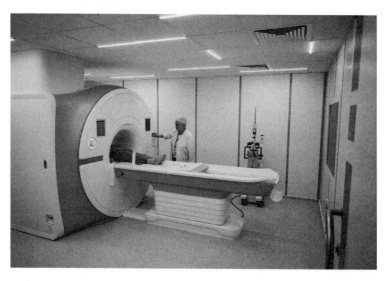

FIGURE 2.1 MRI machine.
Image courtesy of Can Do MS.

The MRI scan provides detailed pictures of the brain and spinal cord. Instead of radiation, the MRI uses a strong magnetic field and computer-generated radio frequency pulses to identify normal and abnormal tissue based on the water content in the tissues (Figure 2.2).

If abnormalities appear in the MRI images, the **radiologist** and MS care provider will determine whether the abnormalities are typical of MS or some other condition. Not all white spots that show up on a brain MRI are due to MS, however. A long list of conditions, ranging from migraine headaches to stroke, can cause changes that will appear on an MRI. Typical MS lesions (see Chapter 1) are round or oval in shape, situated next to and oriented perpendicular to large fluid-filled structures called **lateral ventricles** or at the juncture where the **white matter** and **gray matter** of the brain meet.

MS lesions that appear on MRI indicate that inflammation and damage to the myelin coating around nerve fibers (**demyelination**) have occurred.

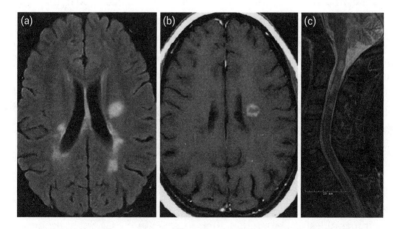

FIGURE 2.2 MRI of the brain and spinal cord with abnormalities consistent with MS. (A) Fluid attenuated inversion recovery (FLAIR) image of the brain with multiple white matter lesions consistent with MS. (B) T1 image with gadolinium (contrast) showing an enhancing brain lesion. (C) Spinal cord image with multiple lesions consistent with MS.

Gadolinium, a **contrast agent**, may be used to identify active inflammation. Gadolinium, which is injected into a vein, causes a feeling of warmth throughout the body. Normally, gadolinium does not get into the brain and is not seen on an MRI. In MS, a lesion that is actively inflamed will take up the gadolinium and appear as a bright spot on certain MRI images. While helpful for identifying new areas of MS activity, gadolinium is not needed for every MRI.

In rare instances, a person who is eventually diagnosed with MS has an initial MRI that appears normal. However, if a person continues to have normal MRI scans, the diagnosis is highly unlikely to be MS.

The 2017 criteria used to diagnose MS (see the section titled "2017 McDonald Diagnostic Criteria") allow the diagnosis of MS to be made, even if a person has only had one attack, if the MRI shows the presence of inflamed and non-inflamed lesions at the same time, or if certain abnormalities are present in their spinal fluid. In other words, the second attack is not required to make the diagnosis as long as the MRI findings confirm that the damage has occurred in different locations at different points in time (separation in time and separation in space; see above).

Because MS is not the only condition that can cause nerve damage and white spots on an MRI, it may sometimes be difficult to identify an MS lesion from one that is caused by another process. A new MRI measure, the number or percentage of lesions that show a **central vein sign** or small hole within the plaque, is emerging as a helpful means of distinguishing MS lesions from lesions caused by other conditions.

The number of lesions varies among individuals with MS, but multiple lesions are expected. In many cases, it is not necessarily the number of lesions but, rather, their location in the CNS that produces symptoms and impairments.

While the list of diseases that can cause spots in the brain is very long, the list of processes that cause damage to both the brain and spinal cord is much shorter, which makes spinal cord imaging very important as well. The presence of spinal cord lesions can often help satisfy the "rules" for diagnosing MS. They may also help in predicting a person's prognosis and guiding treatment.

When a healthy person has an MRI brain scan—for example, following a car accident or for unexplained headaches—and the scan shows evidence of lesions similar to those seen in MS, but they have no MS symptoms or other neurological findings, they are considered to have a radiologically isolated syndrome (RIS). A person with RIS is closely monitored with follow-up MRI scans and neurologic evaluations because approximately 50% of people with RIS go on to develop MS.

Sara is a healthy 35-year-old woman. She is married with two small children and holds a full-time job. One morning as she is toweling off after her shower, she notices numbness in her right leg. Over the next 2 days, the numbness spreads first to her other leg and then moves upward to include her hips. By the fourth day, the numbness reaches to her waist. She also feels a sensation of heaviness in her legs, but the sensation does not interfere with her ability to walk or other usual activities.

When the numbness persists for more than a week, Sara decides to go to the local urgent care. The provider orders an MRI of the brain and spinal cord that shows a single spinal cord lesion. In the absence of any other cause, Sara is considered to have a clinically isolated syndrome (CIS). The urgent care provider recommends a local neurologist who can do additional MRIs and a full neurologic exam. The neurologist starts Sara on a DMT, even though she has not yet met the criteria for MS. Many of the MS DMTs have received U.S. Food and Drug Administration approval for use in CIS based on clinical trials demonstrating a delay in additional symptoms and MRI activity in a person with CIS.

One year later, Sara experiences double vision and fatigue. A follow-up MRI shows additional lesions in the brain, which confirms her diagnosis of MS. The neurologist recommends a change in her DMT in an effort to limit further disease activity.

Lumbar Puncture

A **lumbar puncture** (**spinal tap**) is a procedure in which a sample of **cerebrospinal fluid** (**CSF**), a clear fluid that surrounds the brain and spinal cord, is taken for examination.

Spinal fluid in a person with MS may show certain abnormalities that can help the neurologist make a correct diagnosis. The autoimmune attack on myelin and other tissues in the CNS may result in abnormal antibody production in the spinal fluid, which is measured by the presence of certain immune proteins known as **oligoclonal bands** in the CSF. A "suspicious" lumbar puncture does not definitively point to MS because oligoclonal bands are found in conditions other than MS—which explains why ruling out these other conditions is part of the process for diagnosing MS. Conversely, up to 10% of people with confirmed MS have normal spinal fluid. So, if all the other findings are consistent with an MS diagnosis, normal CSF does not negate the diagnosis.

In many instances, a diagnosis of MS is made without performing a CSF examination; however, a lumbar puncture may be done to provide more evidence of MS when there is insufficient information from other tests and examinations.

Evoked Potentials

Evoked potentials, also called "**evoked responses**," show how nerves respond to various types of stimuli: visual (e.g., a flashing light), auditory (e.g., a click or tone), or sensory (e.g., an electrical pulse to the arm or leg).

Using electrodes pasted to the head, each type of response is detected by recording the brain waves generated when the stimulus is presented. Normally, nerve impulses are transmitted from one point to another in the spinal cord and brain without interruption. MS plaques may slow or block that transmission, so a prolonged or absent evoked potential response indicates nerve damage.

Slowed responses may provide evidence of demyelination in specific parts of the CNS that may not show up on the history, neurologic examination, or MRI. Therefore, they are very useful for detecting clinically silent lesions (areas of nerve damage that do not produce symptoms) or those too small to be seen on an MRI. When the evoked potentials provide evidence of a clinically silent lesion that is the second area of nerve damage in the CNS, this helps fulfill the "rule" for diagnosing MS that requires damage in two distinct areas of the CNS.

Blood Tests

There is currently no single blood test that can diagnose MS, although this is an active area of investigation. Your provider will order a number of blood tests to rule out other conditions that can produce symptoms similar to those seen in MS. Your blood is examined for evidence of certain infections, vitamin deficiencies, other inflammatory diseases such as lupus, and certain metabolic and inherited diseases. There are also blood tests that help diagnose two related demyelinating conditions, NMOSD and MOGAD.

An emerging blood test that measures certain proteins called **neurofilament light chains**, which are produced when axons are damaged, is proving useful in tracking disease activity and response to therapy after diagnosis.

Putting the Picture Together

With the results of the medical history, neurologic exam, and tests, your provider will put all of the evidence together to determine whether you or your family member has MS. The diagnostic criteria for MS help MS care providers make an accurate and timely diagnosis.

2017 McDonald Diagnostic Criteria

Because there is no one definitive test for diagnosing MS, MS experts use the 2017 version of guidelines known as the **McDonald criteria**, named after Ian McDonald, the lead author on the 2001 diagnostic criteria. These criteria give fairly specific rules for using the history, neurologic examination, MRI, CSF findings, and evoked potentials to produce a diagnosis.

New criteria allow certain MRI and CSF findings to fulfill the requirement for separation in time and space on a single MRI. These findings can also make it possible for some people to be diagnosed with MS after only one attack, without having to wait for an additional episode, neurologic symptoms, or repeated MRIs. But the basic principles are the same: There has to be documented evidence of damage to the brain, spinal cord, or optic nerve in more than one place, that occurred at two different time points, with no other disease process being able to account for the findings.

Researchers are also trying to identify **biomarkers** (substances or cells in the brain, blood, or spinal fluid that may appear early in the disease and/or MRI findings that are more specific for MS) so that the diagnosis can be made as quickly and accurately as possible.

Summary

While no single "surefire" test exists to diagnose MS, there are well-established guidelines, and in most cases a diagnosis is made within a few days to a few months. Accurate diagnosis is important so that the appropriate treatment can be started, whether for MS or for another condition that has been identified. Diagnostic methods continue to improve; for example, MRIs are much more sensitive now than they were a decade ago, and much research is being devoted to finding markers that are more sensitive and specific for MS to make the diagnostic process easier and faster for both patients and physicians.

CHAPTER 3

Comprehensive Care of Multiple Sclerosis Over the Lifetime

In this chapter, you will learn:

- What comprehensive care is and why it is important
- The goals of multiple sclerosis care
- Multiple sclerosis disease-modifying therapies(DMTs)
- Multiple sclerosis relapses and how they are treated
- An overview of multiple sclerosis symptom management

If you have recently been diagnosed with multiple sclerosis (MS), you likely have many questions about how the disease is treated and symptoms are managed. We discuss these questions and more, helping you learn about being healthy and well with MS, and introduce you to the members of the MS health care team.

Comprehensive Approach to Multiple Sclerosis Care

Currently, there is no cure for MS; however, treatments and management strategies have evolved significantly so that the disease process can be modified and the symptoms managed effectively.

When we think about MS care over the lifetime, there are five major goals:

1. Maintain and improve overall health and well-being
2. Limit new MS inflammation and damage

3. Treat relapses
4. Manage symptoms
5. Maintain independence and achieve maximal physical, mental, and social function

Reaching these goals is possible with you, your support partner(s), and your MS team working together. One health care professional does not have the expertise to optimally manage all the issues that may arise over the course of your lifetime. Different types of health care professionals will likely be needed. Ideally, the various health care professionals and you will work together in a coordinated approach to help you reach your goals—an approach known as **comprehensive MS care.**

Comprehensive care considers the whole person and all their needs, not just the medical and physical ones. According to the National Multiple Sclerosis Society, the model of comprehensive MS care involves the expertise of many different health care professionals, each contributing in a unique way to the management of the disease and the symptoms it can cause. Sometimes this team works within a single center, while in other cases multiple providers in a community may be involved. In either case, you are at the center of care and the goal is coordinated care to manage the disease, symptoms, and promote comfort a function, independence, health, and wellness (Figure 3.1).

Accessing health care professionals who can help you with specific needs can be challenging based on the availability of the professionals in your area and the cost of care. Various nonprofit organizations (see Appendix 2) and your local hospital, health insurance provider, neurologist, and primary care provider can help you identify health care professionals who can be of help to you. In addition to local health care professionals, many services are available through telemedicine, which can increase your access to additional health care professionals.

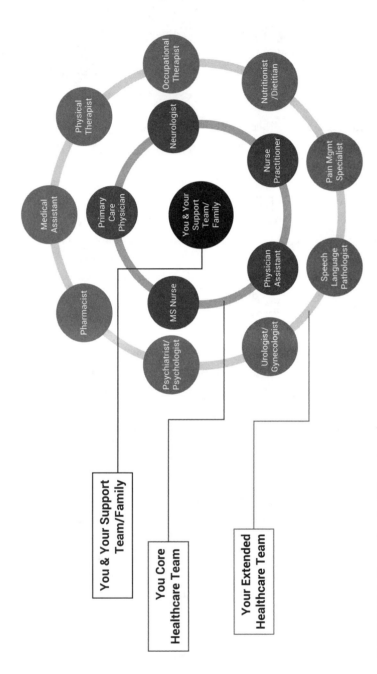

FIGURE 3.1 Comprehensive MS care team.

Goal 1: Maintain and Improve Overall Health and Well-Being

Right now, MS may be your biggest concern, but your overall health is equally important, including attention to preventive health activities, mental health, and healthy lifestyle behaviors. Research has demonstrated that reducing the risks of chronic illnesses such as high blood pressure, heart disease, obesity, and diabetes can positively affect the course of your MS. Mental health issues such as **depression** and **anxiety** (see Chapter 7) are more common in people with MS than the general population and can negatively impact other symptoms, reduce adherence to medical advice, challenge relationships, and reduce overall quality of life. Healthy lifestyle behaviors such as smoking cessation, healthy diet, regular **physical activity**, and adequate sleep have been associated with reduction in the risk of chronic illnesses, improvements in cognitive function, and improvements in mood. They may also improve the overall course of MS.

Goal 2: Limit New Multiple Sclerosis Inflammation and Damage

Treating the MS disease process wasn't possible until 1993, when the first disease-modifying therapy (DMT) was approved by the U.S. Food and Drug Administration (FDA). Since that time, more than 20 DMTs have been FDA-approved. These treatments have been proven in well-designed clinical trials to limit new disease activity (inflammation and nerve damage); reduce the occurrence of new relapses; and, with many of the DMTs, delay or slow disease progression.

Multiple sclerosis DMTs have changed the natural history of MS and improved long-term outcomes. Research has indicated that the number of early relapses and early changes seen on magnetic resonance imaging (MRI) are predictive of the level of disability that can occur over time. While these predictors are not always 100% accurate, most MS specialists and researchers agree that early intervention to manage this disease activity is better than waiting to begin treatment. Newer research suggests that early treatment with more effective agents may also result in better long-term outcomes.

Multiple sclerosis DMTs differ in how they are administered; self-injected, oral, and infused treatments are currently available (Table 3.1). There are different classes of MS treatments, and each class modifies the MS disease process in a unique way by targeting immune system cells and processes, and limiting new inflammation and damage. However, each class of DMT has different side effects and risks associated with their use. (See Appendix 1 for more information about MS DMTs.)

Shared decision-making can help you manage the complexities of choosing the optimal treatment. While you probably don't feel

TABLE 3.1 Multiple Sclerosis Disease-Modifying Therapies[a]

Self-Injected DMTs	Oral (by Mouth) DMTs	Infused (in a Vein) DMTs
Glatiramer acetate	Oral fumarate	Adhesion molecule blocker
Copaxone, Glatopa, glatiramer acetate for injection	Tecfidera, Vumerity, Bafiertam	Tysabri
Interferons	S1P receptor modulators	B cell depleting
Avonex, Betaseron, Extavia, Rebif, Plegridy	Gilenya, Mayzent, Ponvory, Zeposia	Ocrevus, Briumvi
B cell depleting	B and T cell inhibitor	Immunosuppressant
Kesimpta	Aubagio	Lemtrada
	B and T cell depletor	
	Cladribine	

[a]See Appendix 1 for additional information about each FDA-approved DMT.
DMTs, disease-modifying therapies.

qualified to make decisions on your own, you and your MS care provider each have something important to contribute to the process:

- You know yourself—your MS and your goals, fears, concerns, values, and preferences.
- Your MS provider has knowledge of the different treatments, including benefits and risks, and understands the MS disease process. This means that your expertise and experience and the provider's expertise and experience are equally relevant and important in decision-making.
- When you and your MS provider are deciding on a DMT, having information about the treatments can help you
  - understand the treatment options and have confidence in your decision;
  - manage any side effects and risks; and
  - be consistent and persistent with taking the treatment.

The MS DMTs

The MS DMTs are powerful medications, and as such, they have side effects and risks. For example, certain DMTs will impact the types of vaccinations that you can receive and/or when you can receive the vaccinations. And certain DMTs, taken by men or women, can harm an unborn baby. Some are not safe if you are breastfeeding. Talking with your MS provider about the benefits and the risks of the DMTs will help you feel more confident with your decision and better able to manage side effects and persist with the treatment.

Regular follow-up visits with your MS provider are highly recommended to monitor MS disease activity and address any side effects you may be experiencing.

Before beginning the use of DMTs, here are questions to ask your MS provider:

- What will happen if I do not take a DMT or decide to wait before starting one?

- What should I expect from the DMTs? Will my symptoms improve? Will the spots in my brain go away? Will I get worse?
- With so many medications available to treat MS, how will we decide which one is best for me?
- If I want to get pregnant in the near future, how does that impact my treatment options?
- I want to take the medication that is right for me, but I am worried about side effects and risks. Can you explain the trade-offs to me?
- I have heard that certain MS DMTs reduce the effectiveness of vaccinations. Can you please tell me more about that?
- What kinds of tests do I need before I start the DMT, and do I need testing after I start the medication? How often?
- How often does someone on a DMT get MRIs?
- How long do I need to be on a DMT?
- How do we know the DMT is working, and what do we do about it if we decide that it is not working?
- Are all DMTs covered by insurance? Are there programs and resources to help with the cost of the medications?

Some DMTs are considered to be stronger or more effective than others; these are known as **high-efficacy DMTs**. This means that based on their clinical trial results, they have more disease-limiting impact, which translates to less new inflammation, fewer relapses, and more impact on progression of disease. The high-efficacy DMTs are generally considered to be alemtuzumab (Lemtrada), cladribine (Mavenclad), natalizumab (Tysabri), ocrelizumab (Ocrevus), ofatumumab (Kesimpta), and ublituximab (Briumvi). Based on their clinical trial results, some MS researchers also include the **S1P receptor modulators** in the high-efficacy DMT group, and these include fingolimod (Gilenya), ozanimod (Zeposia), ponesimod (Ponvory), and siponimod (Mayzent).

There are certain features of MS and individual characteristics that are indicators that the MS disease course could be more severe.

These characteristics may be considerations for using high-efficacy DMTs early in the disease course. These include the following:

- Younger age at MS onset
- Male sex
- Black or Hispanic/Latinx
- Other illnesses or conditions at the time of MS diagnosis, such as high blood pressure, diabetes, or other cardiac conditions
- High disease activity early in the course of MS (frequent relapses or MRI evidence of disease)
- Incomplete recovery from relapses
- Evidence of MS in the spinal cord early in the disease course

It is reasonable to ask whether everyone with MS should be prescribed a high-efficacy DMT. MS varies from one person to another, and treatment must be determined for each person based on many factors: the individual's disease activity, amount of damage, individual risk tolerance, and individual goals. Take time to think through your own priorities, tolerance for risk (as some high efficacy DMTs have higher risks), personal goals, and ability to manage side effects, and consider talking it over with your care partner. All these things deserve discussion with your MS provider when you are deciding on the right DMT for you.

Goal 3: Treatment of Multiple Sclerosis Relapses

An MS relapse (also known as an exacerbation, attack, or flare) is defined as a new or newly worsening symptom or symptoms of MS that last at least 24 hours and are not associated with an infection or a fever. Relapses occur when there is an area of MS inflammation within the CNS that disrupts nerve transmission and produces one or more symptoms. Symptoms might be a new change in vision, strength, balance, sensation, thinking, speech, or others. Relapses tend to appear over a few days, last for several weeks or even months, and then settle down—either partially or completely. Sometimes a return of old symptoms or worsening of current symptoms can feel like a relapse. When these symptoms are caused by a known trigger such as infection or heat exposure—and not new inflammation—they are known as **pseudoexacerbations** (also called **pseudorelapses**). These types of symptoms are not an actual relapse and will often settle down over a few hours to days.

Pseudorelapses are treated by removing the precipitating factor—by cooling down or treating the infection, for example. Relapses can be treated with steroid medications called **corticosteroids**. These steroid medications that reduce inflammation are completely different from the type of steroid used to build muscle. Corticosteroids are used to treat many conditions, such as allergic reactions, asthma, other autoimmune conditions, and MS relapses. In MS, corticosteroids are given in a high dose over several days (either infused into a vein or taken by mouth in pill form). Corticosteroids have been found to accelerate relapse recovery; however, they do not have any impact on the long-term MS disease process. If the corticosteroids are not effective for the MS relapse, other options are available, including **plasmapheresis** (also called **plasma exchange** or **PLEX**) and **intravenous immunoglobulin (IVIG)**.

Plasmapheresis is a procedure that can be used to treat a relapse and is generally used when steroids cannot be used or are ineffective. Plasmapheresis is used to remove proteins from the **plasma** (the liquid part of the blood) that are thought to contribute to inflammation in the CNS. During the procedure, small amounts of blood are removed through a catheter that has been placed in a large vein. A machine separates the plasma from the blood cells, and a plasma substitute is infused with the cells back into the vein. This procedure is usually done in a hospital or infusion clinic setting. The procedure is repeated over the course of several days.

IVIG can also be used to treat a relapse that has not responded to steroids. In this procedure, antibodies are infused into a vein to help in recovery from a relapse.

As a reminder, DMTs limit new inflammation and therefore new relapses, but they do not treat an existing relapse. Most of the DMTs are approved by the FDA to treat relapsing-remitting MS and active secondary progressive MS (progression with relapses or inflammation seen on MRI). One, ocrelizumab (Ocrevus), is also approved for primary progressive MS. The effect of these medications on reducing relapses is much greater than their effect on disease progression. DMTs that will more effectively slow or halt progression are currently being developed.

Goal 4: Treatment of Multiple Sclerosis Symptoms

Multiple sclerosis DMTs are effective at modifying the MS disease process, but they cannot cure MS or completely stop the disease process. You will still experience neurological symptoms during your lifetime with MS. Different symptoms may come and go, and some will become persistent. And those that are persistent may worsen over time.

Symptoms of MS occur based on the location and extent of inflammation and damage that are disrupting messages within the CNS. In general, treatment of any MS symptom requires a multifocal approach. Medications may be used along with **rehabilitation** strategies (e.g., **physical therapy**, **occupational therapy**, and **speech–language therapy**), **psychotherapy**, **lifestyle modifications**, and other interventions depending on the symptom and its impact on function.

Kirsten has been living with MS for 10 years. She experiences weakness in her right leg that makes walking difficult. The weakness has worsened over the past year or so, and she has recently had multiple trips and near falls, and several complete falls, to the point where she is afraid to go out. Her back hurts because she has been swinging her right leg to avoid tripping.

Kirsten is tearful as she explains her situation and says her MS is making her life miserable. She is grief-stricken, lonely, and missing out on the things that she wants to do. She and her MS care provider discuss the leg weakness and plan a management strategy. They also discuss Kirsten's mood as Kirsten seems to be very down. Her treatment plan includes a prescription for a medication called dalfampridine, which improves walking for some people with MS. The pharmacist counsels Kirsten on the side effects and risks of dalfampridine.

Kirsten is also referred to physical therapy for evaluation and treatment of her mobility issues, and she is referred to a **psychologist** *to address her mood. The* **physical therapist (PT)** *identifies weakness in certain muscles in her right leg and initiates exercises for muscle strengthening. The PT also recommends that Kirsten use a cane to reduce tripping, normalize her* **gait,** *and improve her walking speed. Finally, she is taught exercises to do at home, including specific exercises to do in between PT visits and after her PT is completed.*

Kirsten sees her psychologist regularly to address her mood.

Sometimes different strategies must be tried before the symptoms are managed adequately and may not be as straightforward as in Kirsten's case. However, her case does illustrate multiple strategies to manage her mobility issues, and it illustrates the health care professionals who are needed on her comprehensive care team, including her neurology provider, the pharmacist, the PT, and the psychologist.

Goal 5: Maintaining Independence

Current treatments have been found to reduce the number of people who develop progressive disease. Many people who are diagnosed with MS will maintain complete independence throughout their lifetime. They will continue to work, raise families, and participate in different social and leisure activities. They may have symptoms that cause challenges, but independence is maintained.

However, despite best efforts, some people will have symptoms that persist and a disease that worsens over time. Rehabilitation strategies can help people return to independent function and help them get back, keep, or improve abilities that they need for daily life. These abilities may be physical, emotional, and/or cognitive. Thus, rehabilitation professionals are from a wide range of professions, including physical therapy, occupational therapy, speech–language pathology, psychiatry, psychology, recreation therapy, and many more.

The goals of rehabilitation are individualized and based on each person's situation and challenges. Overall, the goals are to optimize safety and restore function and independence. When you meet with a **rehabilitation specialist**, you will be asked about your goals for rehabilitation. Following an assessment, you and the rehabilitation provider will develop a plan specific to your needs. The plan will be revisited and revised as needed during the course of your rehabilitation therapy. Returning to independence may require a different approach to daily activities or may require an assistive device for independent and safe mobility. You and the rehabilitation specialist will develop the most useful strategies for your specific challenges.

In Chapters 4–9, in which we discuss specific symptoms, more will be presented about rehabilitation and rehabilitation specialists. In addition, brief descriptions of various specialists are provided in the Glossary.

Summary

Multiple sclerosis is a disease that requires a comprehensive approach to care. Multiple specialists may be needed across your lifetime to help you manage the disease process and symptoms. In addition, attention to your overall health and wellness will contribute to how you feel and may also impact the MS disease process.

A collaborative relationship with your neurology provider in which your goals, values, and preferences are considered equally with the neurologist's knowledge of MS and treatments—known as **shared decision-making**—will have a positive impact on your adherence, confidence, and disease outcomes.

DMTs are considered a proven strategy for modifying the MS disease process. More than 20 different treatments are currently available, making the landscape robust and complex. For more information about DMTs, visit the Can Do MS, National Multiple Sclerosis Society, and Multiple Sclerosis Association of America websites. Also, each drug manufacturer has information and resources that can be of help to you.

Section 2

Symptoms of
Multiple Sclerosis

CHAPTER 4

Multiple Sclerosis–Related Fatigue

In this chapter, you will learn:

- What "primary multiple sclerosis fatigue" is
- What additional factors contribute to a person's feelings of fatigue
- How to diagnose, treat, and manage fatigue issues
- How to communicate about it with others

Fatigue is the most common multiple sclerosis (MS) symptom and the one that many people describe as their most challenging and disabling. It is one of the two main causes, along with cognitive challenges (discussed in Chapter 7), of early departure from the workforce.

People with MS describe their fatigue in very graphic terms: "It's like swimming through quicksand . . . wearing weights on my arms and legs . . . lying down under a lead blanket . . . having an empty gas tank 24/7." The imagery is vivid, but the reality is that MS fatigue is invisible. Health care providers, family members, friends, or colleagues can't simply look at a person with MS and assess their fatigue level. And having never experienced a similar type of fatigue, they can't imagine what it feels like. As a result, others may not understand why a person experiencing MS fatigue can no longer do all the things they once did. They may conclude that the person is simply lazy or unmotivated. MS-related fatigue thus contributes to difficulties both at home and at work.

Sharon was diagnosed with MS last year when she was 34 years old. She was referred to the neurologist because she was having a funny "vibrating" feeling down her back when she bent her neck forward. When the neurologist was taking her history, Sharon remembered that for the past 6 months she had felt unusually tired. Her routine had not changed much in her very busy life, with both professional and family responsibilities, and she was sleeping throught the night. Nonetheless, she had been waking up feeling exhausted, and the fatigue only got worse as the day went on. When the neurologist eventually diagnosed Sharon with MS, she told Sharon that the new fatigue was most likely her first MS symptom.

"It seems to come from nowhere," Sharon explains. "I'll get this overwhelming wave of tiredness. It's like I weigh a thousand pounds and just can't do any more. My partner is trying to understand but she just doesn't get it."

What Is Primary Multiple Sclerosis Fatigue?

Unlike other MS symptoms that occur because of inflammation and damage to specific pathways, the source of **primary MS fatigue** is not quite as clear. There are several theories on the cause of MS fatigue:

- The overall activation of the immune system with the release of inflammatory chemicals.
- The recruitment of additional areas of the brain to carry out tasks that damaged areas of the brain can no longer do.
- An overall reduction in nerve transmission throughout the central nervous system.

This type of fatigue may be a person's only MS symptom, or it may be one of many. It can occur in people who have no other physical disability as well as in those with severe disability. Primary MS fatigue can come on suddenly at any time, even after awakening from a good night's sleep, but tends to worsen as the day goes on. Whether engaged in physical activity or a task requiring intense concentration, a person may abruptly "hit a wall" and feel unable to continue without a period of rest.

Secondary Fatigue

Identifying your symptoms as primary MS fatigue can be challenging because so many additional factors can play a role. For example, **secondary MS fatigue** can result from other MS symptoms or the negative effects of those symptoms, as well as medication side effects, **deconditioning**, and other medical conditions. These secondary causes need to be identified and addressed to make a correct diagnosis and manage a person's fatigue most effectively.

Disrupted sleep is common in people with MS. Primary **sleep apnea**, **insomnia**, and **restless leg syndrome** are all more common in people with MS than in the general population. In addition, an overactive bladder, pain, spasms caused by spasticity, and depression and anxiety can all interfere with a good night's sleep.

Medication side effects can make people feel sleepy or tired. It's common for people with MS to be taking several different medications to help manage symptoms, and many of these can make a person feel tired. Among the disease-modifying therapies, beta-interferons are the ones most likely to produce fatigue. Other classes of medications that can produce fatigue include antispasticity agents (baclofen and tizanidine), medications that are used to treat pain (e.g., gabapentin, pregabalin, carbamazepine, and amitriptyline), some antidepressants (including serotonin-reuptake inhibitors such as escitalopram, paroxetine, and fluoxetine), allergy medications such as antihistamines, and even some blood pressure medications. Medication side effects, including fatigue, are one of the reasons for making sure your doctor always has a complete list of your prescription and over-the-counter medications.

Deconditioning also contributes to fatigue. When people become less active in their daily lives and engage in fewer physical activities, their muscles become weaker, and their joints become less flexible. This, in turn, means that moving takes more effort and energy, which makes carrying out everyday tasks more tiring and more challenging.

Dietary choices can also contribute to fatigue. For example, foods high in carbohydrates—particularly simple carbohydrates such as sugar and refined (white) grains—cause a spike in energy followed by feelings of fatigue. Foods that are high in fat are slower to digest, which can slow your ability to use the energy in those foods. Severe and daily caloric restriction will increase fatigue. Alcohol, particularly in significant quantities, can cause sleep disruptions that can contribute to fatigue. And caffeine, while providing a boost of wakefulness, will cause more feelings of exhaustion if consumed in large quantities.

Other medical conditions can also cause or worsen fatigue, including **anemia, thyroid dysfunction**, and infections.

In order to help you manage your fatigue effectively, it's essential for your provider to assess all of these possible factors. Keeping a sleep and activity diary for 2–4 weeks, in which you track your sleep (and everything that interrupts it) as well as your fatigue pattern over the course of each day (when the fatigue starts, when you feel most energized, and when you feel most tired), can help you and your provider identify the sources of your fatigue and the best ways to manage it.

How Is Multiple Sclerosis Fatigue Treated?

Managing fatigue is a three-step process that includes identifying and addressing each of the contributing factors described above, making lifestyle modifications to reduce fatigue, and using medication when needed.

Addressing the Factors Contributing to Fatigue

Once you and your provider have identified each of the issues that may be contributing to your fatigue, it's essential to tackle them one by one. It will likely require a multidisciplinary approach:

- Primary care physician to address other health conditions
- Neurologist and pharmacist to assist with medication side effects
- Neurologist, physical therapist, and/or pain specialist to manage pain that interferes with sleep and daily activities
- Mental health professional to diagnose and treat mood issues that are interfering with sleep
- Occupational therapist to help with energy conservation strategies and environmental modifications and adaptations
- Physical therapist to help with strengthening and conditioning
- **Sleep specialist** to diagnose and manage any existing sleep disorder and provide recommendations for improved sleep habits
- **Urologist** to diagnose and treat and bladder symptoms that may be waking you up night

Making Lifestyle Modifications

Many **lifestyle factors** impact your energy level, including diet, physical activity, heat exposure, and environmental demands.

Eating a healthy, balanced diet filled with colorful fruits and vegetables, whole grains, lean proteins, healthy fats, and limited quantities of salt, added sugars, refined grains, and saturated fats helps reduce fatigue and increase energy. A licensed **nutritionist**, registered dietician, or **health coach** can advise you on diet strategies to meet your needs and potentially increase your energy level.

Inactivity is a major contributor to fatigue. Although it may seem counterintuitive, the best way to increase your energy is to move more. A physical therapist can prescribe a personalized exercise plan that meets your needs and abilities. Some personal trainers also have experience with MS and can help design exercise plans. A complete exercise regimen includes strength training, aerobics, stretching, balance, and posture training, all of which are possible whether you are standing or seated. Lifestyle physical activities—such as dressing and grooming, cleaning, cooking, taking a walk, shopping, or mowing the lawn—can all be tailored to accommodate any limitations you have. A physical therapist or occupational therapist can recommend tools and adaptive equipment to make activities you enjoy accessible and safe for you.

Skier Jimmie Heuga won an Olympic bronze medal in 1964 and was diagnosed with MS in 1970. At that time, doctors advised him to avoid physical activity because it was thought to worsen MS symptoms. In contrast to these long-held assumptions, a significant body of research—beginning with a study inspired by Heuga's beliefs about the value of exercise—has shown that in general, people with MS not only tolerate exercise well but also find that it improves their symptoms and the quality of their lives. The benefits of exercise for people with MS, including those with mild, moderate, or severe disability, are improved physical strength, muscle tone, balance, and coordination, as well as aid in counteracting depression. By contrast, lack of exercise and physical activity can lead a person with MS-related fatigue into a downward spiral of increased fatigue, deconditioning, and depression. Heuga created and followed an exercise regimen for himself that he continued throughout his lifetime.

The majority of people with MS experience heat sensitivity. Engaging in exercise or physical activity can cause the body's core temperature to rise. A person who is heat-sensitive may experience a temporary worsening of neurologic symptoms (similar to what happens when they have a fever due to infection or are in a hot or humid environment). These temporary symptoms are not MS relapses (see Chapter 1), and they don't indicate any new nerve damage or harm. Once the body's temperature returns to normal, the symptoms gradually improve. Using cooling strategies (cooling vests, neck wraps, bandanas, and drinking cold water) during physical activities can help prevent any symptoms—including fatigue—from worsening.

The environment in which a person lives and works has a direct impact on their fatigue level. The more stairs there are to climb, the more bending and reaching required to carry out tasks, and the longer the distance from one room to another, the greater the energy expenditure required. Occupational therapists are experts at helping people modify their environments—particularly kitchens, bathrooms, and offices—in ways that help conserve energy. They can recommend tools and devices that help simplify everyday tasks and also mobility aids to reduce the effort required to navigate those environments.

Let the following helpful reminders (often called the 5 P's) from occupational therapists be your guidebook to energy conservation and fatigue management:

- Planning: Thinking ahead about how you want to use your limited energy; doing your most challenging tasks when you feel your best.
- Prioritizing: Making choices about what's most important to you to ensure that you're using your limited energy in ways that meet your needs.
- Pacing: Moving at a slow and steady pace makes the best use of your energy; rest breaks help you recover more quickly; stopping before you hit the wall helps minimize your recovery time following exertion
- Positioning: How you position yourself during a task helps determine how much energy you use. Don't stand when you can sit; don't store your favorite pots and pans in cabinets that

are difficult to reach; use a raised toilet seat to make toileting less tiring.

- Powering along with tools and gadgets: Doing tasks the easy way rather than the difficult way conserves energy. If you have only so much energy over the course of the day, the use of mobility aids and accessibility gadgets helps ensure that you're not wasting precious energy unnecessarily.

"Jim, aged 54 years, has secondary progressive MS. He has always been a hard worker. According to his wife,"

"Jim comes at two speeds, asleep and 100 miles per hour. Some days, he wakes up feeling pretty energetic. On those days, he tries to cram 3 days' worth of work into 1 day. I've tried to get him to pace himself, but he says he wants to get as much done as possible since he doesn't know if he'll feel this good tomorrow."

"Jim admits that when he does this, the "good" day is typically followed by several days of poor energy and a decreased ability to get much done. After describing this pattern to his neurologist, Jim is referred to an occupational therapist to work on energy conservation." Jim says,

"I really didn't want to go to see the therapist, but after some gentle coaxing from my wife, I did. I have to admit, the advice from the therapist has helped me pace myself. I now have fewer days when I'm really wiped out."

Medications

When exercise and environmental modifications aren't providing enough relief for fatigue, medications can be used to help relieve primary **MS fatigue**. Some studies have indicated no benefit or modest benefit from these medications for the treatment of fatigue, but these can still be tried as some individuals will be helped by their use. These medications are used **off-label** for treatment of MS fatigue.

Amantadine (Symmetrel), which was originally introduced in 1964 to stave off influenza, was unexpectedly found to boost energy levels in some people with MS. When amantadine is taken twice daily, about half of those with the disease find it helpful in reducing fatigue. Generally, a person can recognize whether this drug is working within 2–4 weeks. Some find that the effectiveness of amantadine decreases over time. However, taking a several-day break from the drug and then resuming use may enable it to work effectively again. Generally, the risk of side effects with amantadine is low, but it can cause insomnia if taken too late in the day.

Modafinil (Provigil) is a prescription drug that promotes wakefulness and alertness. It was originally developed to treat the neurologic disorder narcolepsy, which is characterized by abnormal and sudden sleepiness. It has also been studied by the military as an alternative to amphetamines in situations in which troops face lengthy periods of sleep deprivation and must remain alert. Several studies examining modafinil's effectiveness for primary MS fatigue have shown that it provides some benefit, whereas others have shown no benefit over a placebo. Modafinil may be taken once or twice daily, but many people report benefit when they use it on an as-needed basis. Like amantadine, it can cause insomnia if taken too late in the day. The risk of side effects is low, but occasionally modafinil can produce jitteriness. In addition, some people experience other side effects, such as headache, nausea, and rapid heart rate. Multiple generic versions of modafinil have helped reduce the cost.

Armodafinil (Nuvigil), which is similar to modafinil, was approved by the U.S. Food and Drug Administration (FDA) in 2007 for the treatment of excessive sleepiness associated with narcolepsy, obstructive sleep apnea, and shift work sleep disorder. This form allows for once-daily dosing but otherwise has the same benefits and potential side effects as modafinil. The availability of generic formulations has helped reduce the cost.

Before armodafinil became available, various prescription stimulants were commonly used to counteract MS-related fatigue, including methylphenidate (Ritalin) and the mixture of amphetamine and dextroamphetamine (Adderall and Strattera). Although both carry the potential for tolerance or addiction, research has shown that this generally does not become a major problem. A 2009 study by the National Institute on Drug Abuse found a low potential for tolerance or addiction when Ritalin was used for medical purposes.

Antidepressant medications may be helpful as well, particularly, of course, when fatigue is associated with depression. Because MS symptoms seem to influence one another, it's not unusual for a person to experience a combination of fatigue, depression, and cognitive problems. Distinguishing between MS-related fatigue and depression-related fatigue can be tricky. People with MS fatigue want to participate in an activity, but their bodies resist going along for the ride. In depression-related fatigue, the desire to participate in activities may be greatly reduced. Fatigue from either source will generally diminish the ability to concentrate, which tends to make cognitive problems seem worse. Because people with MS can have some or all of these problems from time to time, antidepressants (particularly formulations that are more activating) may serve to increase energy and improve both mood and concentration. None of the antidepressants or medications for sleep disorders that are used to treat MS fatigue are FDA-approved for this purpose, which means they are being used off-label. Therefore, in the United States, there may be challenges with insurance coverage.

A Word About Communication

While your fatigue may seem overwhelming and obvious to you, keep in mind that it's invisible to others. And no matter how much they love and care about you, family, friends, and colleagues can't read your mind. Be prepared to describe your fatigue in ways that people can visualize and let them know when and how it's most likely to affect you. Help them understand that your inability to participate in something isn't about them—it's about you—and as soon as you are able, you would like to reschedule your plans or catch up on your work. Using metaphors and signals can be very helpful:

- "I have one dollar's worth of energy to spend when I wake up in the morning and you have 5 dollars' worth. You will likely have energy left after you work all day. But, if I spend too much at one time, I won't have enough left to do other things—which means I must plan and prioritize."
- "Today is a green light [or thumbs up] day, which means I have energy to do at least some of things I want to do" or "Today is a red light [or thumbs down] day and I'm having a lot of fatigue. Can we plan a rain check?"

Summary

Fatigue is a challenge for many people with MS. Fatigue can be a symptom of MS itself or may be due to other causes, such as depression, other medical conditions, disrupted sleep, medication side effects, or deconditioning from lack of activity. Careful assessment of the symptoms is needed to determine the cause of the fatigue so that the most appropriate and useful treatment plan can be developed. As with most symptoms of MS, approaching fatigue management from different angles is most useful. Your health care team can help you manage the factors that contribute to your fatigue, with an exercise regimen, healthy eating, improved sleep, environmental modifications, the use of mobility devices, gadgets and tools, and medications, when needed, all potentially playing a role.

Be prepared to talk about your fatigue with your MS care provider and your family members—what it feels like; when it happens; and what, if anything, helps to relieve it. People have a hard time understanding what they cannot see. Your ability to describe it to others and advocate for your needs will help ensure you get the care and assistance you need.

CHAPTER 5

Mobility Symptoms

In this chapter, you will learn:

- How mobility can be challenged by multiple sclerosis
- The factors that contribute to mobility issues in multiple sclerosis
- Strategies to improve mobility

Our feelings of independence are intertwined with our mobility. When mobility is compromised, we can start to feel restricted, vulnerable, and dependent. Although multiple sclerosis (MS) can affect all aspects of mobility, there are several strategies people with MS can use to improve their mobility and reclaim their function and independence.

Many of the symptoms of MS are invisible to others. You cannot tell just by looking at a person with MS whether they are experiencing fatigue, pain, or cognitive challenges. On the other hand, when someone uses a **mobility aid,** it is clear that their ability to move has been affected. For this reason, it's not surprising that mobility is one of the first issues people with MS want to discuss with their care providers.

Mobility Depends on Many Complex Functions

The good news is that an MS diagnosis doesnt always fast-track you to impaired mobility. Twenty years after diagnosis, approximately two-thirds of people with MS will continue to function independently.

Nonetheless, most people with MS do experience some changes in their mobility—either temporarily during a relapse or more permanently as the disease progresses. Most people take walking and moving their arms for granted, not realizing how many neurological functions are involved in these routine motions. Strength, sensation, coordination, balance, **proprioception** (the ability to detect changes in the body's position in space), and muscle tone all play a role in the ability to move and walk, and MS may affect one or more of them. Let's take a brief look at how each of these functions should operate, how MS can affect them, and what can be done to deal with those effects. More details about the management of each of these functions are provided in the section titled "Addressing Mobility Symptoms."

Strength

At the simplest level, muscles move in response to signals from the brain. MS disrupts or halts signal transmission between the brain and the rest of the body by damaging the myelin insulation around nerve fibers (axons) in the brain and spinal cord, as well as the axons themselves (see Chapter 1).

Weakness can result when the central nervous system (CNS) has difficulty receiving, processing, and sending messages. When this communication is interrupted, changes in function, including mobility, can occur and may be temporary or permanent. For example, a person with MS may find that their strength varies considerably, even over the course of a single day. In the morning, picking up a heavy object may be possible, but in the afternoon, after a long walk or an hour sitting out in the sun, lifting their arms or getting out of a chair is difficult. These changes occur because demyelinated axons that are still able to send messages may shut down temporarily due to overexertion or exposure to excessive heat. Other people may have disruption of axons that is severe enough to stop nerve transmission partially or completely in certain areas of the brain. This can cause changes in function that are persistent and that may worsen over time.

Two muscle groups, the **hip flexors** and **ankle dorsiflexors**, play a major role in walking and are especially susceptible to weakening in MS. The hip flexor muscles help bring the knee toward the abdomen, while the ankle dorsiflexors bring the toes and feet off the ground. Ankle dorsiflexor weakness results in **foot drop**. If a person with foot drop has strong hip flexors, they can raise their knee high enough to avoid dragging their toes. The hip flexors in some people with MS are too weak to enable them to do this, so they compensate by swinging the weak leg out or hiking their hip up on one side to keep their toes from dragging. Hip flexor weakness and/or foot dorsiflexor weakness will increase the chances of falling.

Managing Weakness

A physical therapist can evaluate your gait and strength and recommend an exercise regimen to improve both. The physical therapist can also recommend and demonstrate assistive devices that can help you walk farther (and more safely) with a more normalized gait. Examples of assistive devices include **rollators**, wheelchairs, **ankle–foot orthotics (AFOs)**, and **forearm crutches** (Figures 5.1A–5.1D), as well as canes, **walking poles**, Lofstrand **crutches**, and **hip flexion assist devices (HFADs)** (not shown in the figure, but your physical therapist can provide greater detail and the benefits of their use).

Although a physical therapist can't prescribe medications to help with your weakness, Ampyra (dalfampridine) is a medication that

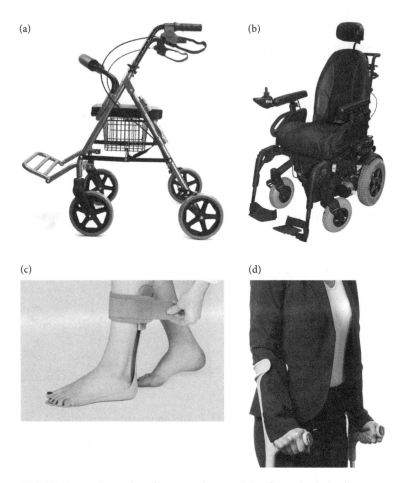

FIGURE 5.1 Examples of assistive devices: (A) a four-wheeled rollator, (B) a custom electric wheelchair, (C) an ankle–foot orthotic (AFO); and (D) a forearm crutch.
(C) Reproduced with permission from Can Do Multiple Sclerosis.

your MS care provider can prescribe to help with muscle strength and walking. Taken by mouth every 12 hours, it can temporarily help the disrupted nerve signals work better, which may improve strength and walking.

Bob has had primary progressive MS for the past 12 years and is now 53 years old. An avid runner, he found that he tended to stumble during longer runs. Over the years, his runs have become shorter because of a tendency to drag his left foot. At the start of a run, he can lift his legs and feet normally, but after approximately half a mile, he begins to drag his left foot and experiences increasing stiffness in his leg. These problems worsen until he believes he must stop or risk falling.

Bob's MS care provider refers him to a physical therapist for a walking evaluation. The physical therapist observes his walking and notices that the toes of Bob's left shoe are more scuffed than those on his right. A left foot drop is diagnosed, and the physical therapist recommends an assistive device called an AFO to help lift Bob's foot and improve his gait. In addition, Bob is shown various exercises to strengthen his ankle and leg. With exercise and a customized AFO, Bob can walk better—and even return to some running.

Balance and Coordination

Demyelination and the resulting formation of scar tissue in the CNS can also produce three symptoms involving muscle movement and coordination: **ataxia**, **tremors**, and **dysmetria**.

Ataxia is a disturbance of balance and coordination. It can occur in the limbs, the trunk, or while walking. For example, a person with walking or gait ataxia will appear unsteady and may stumble from side to side. Ataxia, particularly when it occurs with walking, may be helped with assistive devices such as a rollator, which can help improve gait and prevent falls. A physical therapist can provide exercises to improve balance and may use strategies such as a weighted belt to help compensate for ataxia.

Tremor is an involuntary rhythmic movement of a body part, usually an arm or leg but sometimes the head as well. For tremors in the upper extremities, an occupational therapist can recommend weighted utensils to dampen the tremor for eating, writing, or grooming. Other tools and strategies can be employed for additional activities.

Medications can also be used (off-label) to help with tremors, including Valium-type medications (benzodiazepines) such as diazepam and clonazepam, or some antiseizure medications. These medications may reduce tremors but may also cause sleepiness, and, in the case of benzodiazepines, tolerance and dependence.

Dysmetria is the undershooting and overshooting of an intended movement toward a target—for example, reaching out to shake someone's hand and grabbing their elbow instead.

All three of these symptoms (ataxia, tremor, and dysmetria) can affect mobility. For example, someone whose strength is otherwise normal but who has ataxia or dysmetria (or both) may find walking and other activities difficult because of impaired balance and incoordination.

Danielle was diagnosed with MS 8 years ago and is now 31 years old. She has normal strength in her arms and legs but has difficulty walking because of poor balance. She stumbles frequently and drifts from side to side, resulting in frequent falls. Danielle's MS care provider believes that Danielle would benefit from using an assistive device such as a walker or cane. However, Danielle is opposed to using anything to help her walk because it would mean that she is "giving in" to her MS. Her provider also recommends physical therapy. The physical therapist helps Danielle understand the advantages of using an assistive device: She would be safer and less likely to fall, she would move more confidently, and she would be "taking charge of her MS" rather than giving in to it.

Proprioception: A Sense of Self and the Space Around Us

When we intentionally move our arms or legs, several things happen: The brain sends a signal down the spinal cord to the muscles and joints, telling them what body parts to move, how fast, and in what direction. In response, other parts of the CNS help guide that movement by providing information about how the body is moving and ensuring that our movements are smooth, controlled, and coordinated. And the muscles and joints send signals back to the brain, telling it where the body part that is to be moved is already positioned in space. This latter information is called proprioception or "position sense."

Proprioception gives you essential information about where you and your body parts are in space. Normal functioning of this important sensory function is essential to coordinated movements, balance, and walking. MS can cause significant changes in proprioception, which can have a major impact on your ability to stand, walk, or perform basic activities of daily living, regardless of how strong you are. Humans are top-heavy animals: As we tilt one way or the other, our changes in position are relayed to the brain, which sends out nerve signals that enable us to take corrective action to avoid tipping over. All this happens continuously and outside our awareness.

Multiple sclerosis–related nerve damage that disrupts the transmission of proprioceptive signals to the brain may make a person wobble or tilt so far that a fall is inevitable. People with impaired proprioception due to MS are often thought by unknowing observers to have had too much to drink. They use walls, furniture, or the person next to them to keep steady. When the brain isn't receiving the proprioceptive signals it needs for proper balance, visual information becomes more important. When proprioception is impaired, walking in the dark, not looking straight ahead while walking, or standing with your eyes closed (e.g., when you wash your hair in the shower) all increase your risk of falling.

Managing Impaired Proprioception

Strategies to compensate for impaired proprioception include the use of assistive devices, keeping a night light on at night to maintain visual cues for where you are in space, and looking straight ahead when walking. A physical therapist can assess your proprioception issues and recommend strategies to help you move better and more safely.

Vestibular Symptoms

The **vestibular system** includes the inner ear and the brain. Fluid within specialized canals in the inner ear moves with movement. Sensors in the inner ear communicate this movement to the brain so that we can maintain our balance. In MS, the pathways between the brain and the inner ear can be disrupted and produce symptoms of **vertigo**, **dizziness**, and feeling off balance. These symptoms affect mobility and contribute to falls. A specialized type of rehabilitation, **vestibular rehabilitation** (VRT), can help improve balance. In VRT, exercises are used to help the vestibular system adapt in ways that increase gaze stability and posture stability, reduce symptoms of vertigo, and improve the ability to carry out activities of daily living.

Muscle Tone

Mobility also depends on normal **muscle tone**, which refers to how loose or stiff the muscles are. Muscles can flex or extend, which is what enables body parts to move. With normal muscle tone, there is a balance between the muscles that bend or flex a body part and the muscles that straighten or extend a body part. But as many as 75% of people with MS experience a chronic state of excessive muscle tension or tone, which is called spasticity. Although spasticity tends to persist over time, the degree of spasticity can vary. Spasticity, or increased muscle tone, may occur when a limb is extended away from the body (referred to as increased extensor tone). Your leg may suddenly become locked and refuse to bend, for example, or a limb can simply feel stiff and difficult but not impossible to move.

A sudden tightening of muscles in a leg or around the torso is referred to as a **spasm**. Although spasms are usually brief, they can be painful and recurrent, and they tend to be more frequent during the night (referred to as **nocturnal spasms**). During a spasm, the person may be temporarily unable to straighten a bent limb or bend a straightened limb.

Managing Spasticity

Spasticity can be effectively treated through rehabilitation and with medications, when needed. Regular stretching with specific stretching exercises can reduce spasticity significantly. Stretching while in a non-heated pool creates an environment in which the water helps reduce excess muscle tone.

Several oral medications to discuss with your MS care provider that may help with this symptom include baclofen, tizanidine, diazepam, clonazepam, lorazepam, and cannabinoids. Baclofen comes in several different formulations for oral use and can also be delivered in very small doses into the fluid around the spinal cord through a **baclofen pump,** which is an implanted device that delivers small doses of a specialized formulation of baclofen directly into the spinal fluid in the lower back. For people who cannot tolerate oral baclofen or who are not helped by the oral formulation, a pump can be a viable alternative. Tizanidine is another oral treatment for spasticity. The initial dose is titrated from a small dose to the full dose over several days. Diazepam, clonazepam, and lorazepam are sometimes used for nocturnal spasms because they cause significant drowsiness and last through the night. Cannabinoids are used by many and subjectively seem to reduce spasticity and spasms for some.

All of these medications can be effective for the treatment of spasticity. And each has side effects. So, learning the benefits and risks of these medications can help you make the best decision for you.

Jane was diagnosed with MS 10 years ago and is now 44 years old. Jane experiences spasms in her legs at night, particularly after a busy day that includes extensive walking. She finds that her legs cramp behind her knees during the night, interrupting her sleep. Sometimes, her toes curl and she needs to pry them into a normal position with her hands. Jane reports these symptoms to her MS care provider, who prescribes the medication tizanidine to be taken at bedtime to relieve some of the muscle tightness. In addition, he recommends that she see a physical therapist who can teach her stretching exercises.

Finding the "Right" Amount of Extensor Tone

Everyone needs a certain amount of muscle tone. Too much **extensor tone** in the legs may result in pain and difficulty with mobility, particularly walking. A s**cissoring gait,** which refers to the knees and thighs pressing together or crossing while walking, can also result from high muscle tone or spasticity. However, if MS has also resulted in leg weakness, some increase in extensor tone can help a person stand and walk.

Additional Challenges to Mobility

In addition to the direct causes of mobility challenges, mobility can also be challenged by other MS symptoms and even non-MS conditions.

Fatigue, as noted in Chapter 4, is a common symptom of MS and can affect mobility because there is not enough energy to move. When a person moves less, their muscles get weaker from disuse, which in turn makes mobility even more difficult. Movement is needed for muscles to maintain strength and flexibility. Mood and cognitive symptoms (discussed in greater detail in Chapter 8) can also impact mobility. With low mood or depression, there may be little motivation to "get up and go," and related cognitive symptoms such as slowed processing speed, impaired decision-making, and memory difficulties may further compromise mobility.

If a person with MS has other conditions as well, known as **comorbidities**, this may also make mobility more challenging. Examples include shortness of breath from lung or heart problems, pain in the legs from circulatory issues, and obesity that can make movement more difficult. These issues will also need attention as mobility issues are assessed and managed.

Addressing Mobility Symptoms

Multiple sclerosis can affect mobility by causing muscle weakness, faulty coordination, impaired balance, disrupted proprioception, and spasticity. All these symptoms can be addressed, and potentially alleviated, through physical therapy, assistive devices, and medication, when needed.

Working with a Physical Therapist

A referral to a knowledgeable physical therapist who is familiar with MS is important—even before an individual with MS has mobility or walking problems—so that the most appropriate exercises and training can be prescribed. A physical therapist can recommend exercises that can be useful for maintaining strength and flexibility before mobility problems occur. Then, if problems with increased spasticity or issues with mobility do occur, the individual already has an established physical therapy provider who can modify the treatment plan to meet the new challenges. People who already have mobility problems can work with a physical therapist to identify the contributing factors and develop a personalized set of exercises aimed at improving strength, flexibility, muscle control, and balance. And an individual exercise routine will contain some mixture of stretching, strengthening, balance, and cardiovascular exercises, as well as specific strategies directed at compensating for specific deficits.

The following are important principles to remember when someone with MS exercises:

- While most of us want to be in better shape, the "no pain, no gain" adage will not work in MS. Exercising to the point of exhaustion in MS could produce excessive fatigue, leaving the individual unable to participate in normal daily activities.
- Vigorous exercises can also produce excessive heat in the body, which can cause temporary weakness and fatigue for many living with MS. Thus, developing an exercise plan with a rehabilitation specialist who is knowledgeable about MS will likely produce the best exercise program for each individual.

Making Optimal Use of Assistive Technology

For many people, the primary goal of working with a physical therapist is to walk better. To accomplish this goal, some people with MS will need assistive devices to support their mobility. For some people with MS, the idea of using an assistive device feels like "giving up" or "letting MS win." While this is understandable, assistive devices can also mean triumphing over the limitations of MS. Without an assistive device, some people with MS may find their world getting smaller. They may feel shut out of many enjoyable activities, such as sporting events, family gatherings, and shopping. If a walker or cane allows someone to attend their child's soccer game or their 20th class reunion, that's not a loss; it's a win. Think of an assistive device as the right tool for getting you where you want to go and doing what you need to do, safe from falls and injury.

If you are thinking about starting to use a mobility aid, it's important to seek information and guidance from your MS care provider and physical therapist. Using the appropriate device(s) in the proper way is important. As MS functional abilities can vary from day to day, sometimes several types of assistive devices are necessary. The goal is to develop a tool chest that allows you to engage in the activities that are important to you, whether it's a good day or a not-so-good day. Keep in mind, however, that even a device as simple as a cane should be obtained with a prescription so that you are using the correct type of cane—with the correct height, handle, and base for optimal mobility and safety.

Wheeled Devices

Wheeled devices require an evaluation by a physical therapist, occupational therapist, or **seating and mobility specialist (SMS)** to ensure that the seating, arm or leg rests, cushions, and the weight of the chair are right for you. The physical or occupational therapist or SMS will work collaboratively with your MS care provider to ensure that the prescription is correctly written for the device you need. Motorized devices are very expensive, and while most insurers will cover them, they will not cover multiple motorized devices. Thus, determining the correct device for your current and anticipated needs is very important. Issues to consider include cost, portability, and the ability to maneuver the motorized device inside the home. Devices should never be ordered online without the input and careful evaluation of a rehabilitation specialist familiar with motorized devices.

Devices to Manage Foot Drop

Leg weakness, particularly foot drop, is very common in MS. An ankle-foot orthotic (made by an **orthotist**) has been the usual device used for foot drop. The AFO (see Figure 5.1C) is an L-shaped plastic or light-weight carbon device that fits under the foot and up the back of the weak leg to prevent the foot from "dropping" forward. Thus, during the gait cycle, the toe is prevented from dropping, and tripping is prevented.

Wireless electronic devices that can help normalize the gait in those with foot drop are also available. These devices work by sending an electrical signal to the peroneal nerve in the lower leg that causes the ankle to flex during the gait cycle.

Device to Manage Hip Flexion Weakness

An HFAD may help compensate for hip flexion weakness. The HFAD consists of a belt worn around the waist, with an elastic band that connects the belt to the top of a person's shoe on the affected leg. The tension on the elastic band helps bring the hip up to assist in walking.

Device to Increase Hand Mobility

Electronic devices are available to stimulate nerves in the hand to help restore some function. As with the lower extremity devices, these are not for everyone, but they may be useful tools. Working with your rehabilitation specialist and your MS care provider will help you identify the correct device for you.

Summary

If you are anxious about your walking ability or other mobility issues that could occur due to MS, you are not alone. Nearly everyone with MS worries about potential mobility problems, especially when first diagnosed. It's important to remember that motor problems do not happen to everyone with MS and that when they do occur, many options exist for managing them in a way that allows you to do the things you want to do.

When MS affects walking, it is necessary to ascertain whether muscle weakness, faulty coordination, disrupted proprioception, deconditioning, or spasticity—either singly or in combination—is contributing to the problem. Physical therapy, assistive devices, and medications can all play a role in improving and maintaining mobility. Staying mobile is important to your health, safety, and independence. Look to the members of your health care team to assess the factors that are impacting your mobility and take advantage of the treatments and tools that can help you stay mobile in your everyday life.

CHAPTER 6

Sensory Symptoms

In this chapter, you will learn:

- How multiple sclerosis affects sensation
- How multiple sclerosis affects vision
- How multiple sclerosis affects the "special senses" (taste, smell, and hearing)
- How to treat sensory symptoms

People with multiple sclerosis (MS) may experience a variety of sensory disturbances in parts of their body, including loss of sensation or the presence of abnormal sensations. For a long time, people with MS were told that pain was not a symptom of MS, but today we know that MS can cause many different types of painful sensations.

How Multiple Sclerosis Affects Sensation

As discussed in Chapter 1, the demyelination and nerve damage that occur in MS alter the way electrical signals or messages are transmitted between the body and the central nervous system. This nerve damage not only disrupts or blocks transmission of electrical signals but also can produce cross talk between nerves or a kind of "static." The blocked transmission or static produces sensory abnormalities and a decrease in normal sensory function.

Sensory symptoms may include the blunting of normal sensations (e.g., in the form of numbness) as well as unpleasant sensations, such as burning. Unpleasant, annoying sensations such as numbness, tingling, or "pins and needles" are called **paresthesias**. When the new sensations cause pain or discomfort, they are called **dysesthesias**. Like many MS-related symptoms, paresthesias and dysesthesias are not unique to MS and can often be seen in other medical conditions.

Paresthesias and Dysesthesias

Parasthesias may feel like the following:

- A bug is crawling on one's skin
- A hair is tickling the skin
- Tingling
- A feeling of wetness on the skin
- An itching sensation
- "Pins and needles"

Diane has had MS for 4 years and is now 31 years old. When she was diagnosed, she was experiencing a tingling sensation in her left foot and leg up to the hip. Since that time, she has had a mild tingling sensation in the toes of her left foot. It is not really painful; rather, she describes it as annoying, with some days being worse than others. Sometimes in the evening, when she is very tired or has been on her feet much of the day, she notices more tingling in her toes. Once, about 2 years after her diagnosis, Diane felt discomfort in her toes and at the top of her foot. For a short period, wearing shoes with laces was very uncomfortable and produced a painful electrical sensation in her foot (dysesthesia). This lasted about 2 weeks and then went away, but she now continues to have a constant mild tingling in her toes.

Dysesthesias, a type of **neuropathic pain**, cause more painful types of sensations. The "**MS hug**," which feels like a very tight belt or girdle around the abdomen or torso, signals damage to parts of the spinal cord that transmit messages to those parts of the body. It can cause squeezing or burning sensations that can make activities difficult.

Lhermitte's sign, which is caused by demyelination in the cervical spinal cord (neck), feels like a series of electric buzzing–type sensations that can range from annoying to very painful. The sensations radiate down the spine and/or into the arms or legs when the neck is flexed forward. This symptom may be present for weeks to months and then disappear, only to spontaneously reappear sometime in the future. While Lhermitte's sign can be alarming and uncomfortable, you will not cause any new damage by flexing your neck when you have this symptom.

Trigeminal neuralgia causes facial pain—sometimes quite intense—that travels along one of the three branches of the **trigeminal nerve**, which supplies sensation to the face. The intense, electric shock–like pains may last seconds or minutes. The most common form of this pain, which is felt in the lower two-thirds of the face, can be triggered by chewing or even by a very light touch on the cheek.

Occipital neuralgia causes pain along the **occipital nerve**, which exits the base of the skull and supplies sensation to the scalp. Occipital neuralgia may result in pain ranging from dull to intense, sometimes with hypersensitivity to touch over the scalp.

Burning sensations, such as a sunburn-like feeling or feeling as though one's skin is too close to a flame, are common in MS. And like other pain sensations, they are often worse at night. Electric or stabbing sensations can occur intermittently and, like other pain sensations, can range from mild to intense. These can occur sporadically or, for some people, multiple times throughout the day.

Treating Dysesthesias and Paresthesias

Nerve pain does not respond well to conventional pain medicines such as acetaminophen, anti-inflammatory medications like ibuprofen, or opiates. One very effective non-medication treatment for dysethesias is **cognitive–behavioral therapy (CBT)**. CBT is a type of talk therapy that helps people identify negative thoughts and develop skills to change them and the behaviors that go with them. Because the perception of pain is in the brain, changing negative or catastrophic thoughts about the pain ("This is unbearable . . . it will never go away . . . I can't live with this pain") can change a person's perception of that pain and the behaviors that fuel the perception. This change in perception allows the person to focus on other things, engage in enjoyable activities, and experiment with self-care activities, even though the pain is still present.

Nerve pain is also treated with anticonvulsant or antidepressant medications. Because these medications work by reducing electrical and chemical nerve signals, they are particularly useful for MS pain management. But while they lessen the discomfort of paresthesias or dysesthesias, they do not restore normal sensation. Side effects may include dizziness, drowsiness, unsteadiness, and nausea.

Table 6.1 lists some of the more commonly used medications for uncomfortable **sensory symptoms**, along with their possible side effects. These are not complete lists of side effects, and the risks and benefits of any medication should be discussed with your MS care provider. In almost all cases, these medications are being used off-label when prescribed to treat pain, meaning they are approved by the U.S. Food and Drug Administration to treat conditions other than pain. Sometimes, this poses challenges with insurance coverage.

While antiseizure medications are quite effective in treating trigeminal neuralgia, not everyone will respond to them, and the pain may persist for those taking them to treat this symptom. In such cases, persistent trigeminal neuralgia may need to be treated with a surgical procedure that interrupts the signaling from the trigeminal nerve. A variety of surgical procedures may be used to interrupt the pain signal, but as with any surgical procedure, the risks and benefits should be discussed with the surgeon so that an informed decision can be made.

TABLE 6.1 Medications Used for Dysesthesia

Medication	Side Effects
Antidepressants	
Amitriptyline (Elavil)	Dry mouth, drowsiness, blurred vision, constipation, urinary retention, weight gain
Venlafaxine (Effexor)	Nausea, headache, drowsiness, dizziness, loss of appetite, nervousness, weight gain, sexual dysfunction
Duloxetine (Cymbalta)	Nausea, headaches, drowsiness, dry mouth, dizziness, weight gain, sexual dysfunction
Nortriptyline (Pamelor)	Dry mouth, drowsiness, constipation, urinary retention
Anticonvulsants	
Gabapentin (Neurontin)	Dizziness, drowsiness, coordination problems, swelling in the feet/legs, weight gain
Tiagabine hydrochloride (Gabitril)	Dizziness, weakness, tremor, drowsiness
Pregabalin (Lyrica)	Dizziness, drowsiness, problems with coordination, weight gain
Carbamazepine (Tegretol/ Carbatrol)	Dizziness, drowsiness, unsteadiness, nausea, skin rash, abnormal blood counts (blood tests needed periodically)
Oxcarbazepine (Trileptal)	Headaches, drowsiness, dizziness, unsteadiness, nausea (blood tests needed periodically)
Lamotrigine (Lamictal)	Dizziness, headaches, double vision, coordination problems

Occipital neuralgia can also be treated with antiseizure medications such as carbamazepine, oxcarbazepine, and gabapentin. Anti-inflammatory medications such as indomethacin may also be helpful. Local injections of steroids and anesthetic agents at the base of the skull can be used to both treat and diagnose occipital neuralgia.

Several treatment options are available for small areas of skin affected by uncomfortable sensory changes. An over-the-counter topical ointment containing capsaicin may be helpful. Capsaicin is the chemical that gives hot peppers, such as jalapeños, their spicy kick. When applied to the skin, capsaicin blunts the pain by depleting the nerve endings of the chemical they need to relay painful sensory information to the spinal cord. Capsaicin should not be applied to broken or abraded skin or applied anywhere near the eyes or mouth. Ice packs and/or lidocaine patches (numbing medicine) may also provide effective topical relief.

Dysesthesias that do not respond to any of the treatments discussed above may require referrals to other specialists who can provide alternative treatment options such as acupuncture, pain management, neurosurgery, or integrative medicine.

Musculoskeletal Pain

Multiple sclerosis can also produce **musculoskeletal pain** in the muscles and joints. Musculoskeletal pain is best addressed by a physical therapist, who can provide exercise recommendations, gait training, and instruction in the correct use of mobility aids. Spasticity, or muscle tightness, can be severe enough to be painful. Sometimes, sudden spasms or uncomfortable postures can occur in an arm or leg. Spasticity generally responds to stretching and use of antispasticity agents (see Chapter 5 for more information about spasticity management). When weakness or balance problems cause walking difficulties, people with MS may experience pain caused by poor posture or body alignment, an altered gait, or the incorrect use of assistive devices, any of which can put excess strain on muscles and joints. Common symptoms of these types of poor body mechanics include back or neck pain or other muscle aches. Arm pain caused by leaning on a walker or crutches can also occur.

Vision Changes in Multiple Sclerosis

Visual impairment is common in MS, most often caused by inflammation in the optic nerve (optic neuritis) or in the nerves that control eye movements. Optic neuritis is a temporary loss of vision that most often occurs in one eye at a time. The person may experience a variety of visual difficulties, ranging from a blind spot in the middle of their vision to complete inability to see out of one eye. Most often, this change develops over several hours or days. About 50% of the time, the visual loss is accompanied by painful eye movements. There may also be a change in color vision, in which colors, especially red, appear washed out or gray. Optic neuritis is commonly treated with a brief course of corticosteroids that can accelerate recovery of vision, either fully or partially, in the affected eye. If the steroids are not effective, other treatments, such as intravenous immunoglobulin or plasmapheresis, may be tried.

Optic neuritis is not unique to MS. As mentioned in Chapter 2, there are two other conditions that are similar to MS which commonly cause optic neuritis: neuromyelitis optica spectrum disorder (NMOSD) and myelin oligodendrocyte glycoprotein antibody-associated disorder (MOGAD).

In addition to the optic nerve, clear vision is dependent on intact function of three pairs of nerves that control eye movements (the oculomotor, **trochlear**, and **abducens** nerves). When MS affects the function of any of these nerves, or other parts of the brain that are involved in vision, other visual symptoms may result. The most common are blurred vision, **diplopia** (double vision), and shaky or "jumping" vision (**nystagmus**), which makes the world appear as though it is moving when it is not. When these symptoms happen, they are usually treated as though the person is having an MS exacerbation—with a short course of steroids. Sometimes, other medications are tried, such as antiseizure medications or benzodiazepines. In addition, a referral to a low-vision clinic for remedies such as special lenses may be appropriate.

Hearing

While it is very uncommon for MS to cause problems with hearing, it does occasionally happen. People may experience decreased hearing in one or both ears and/or ringing in the ears (**tinnitus**). Because hearing problems are uncommon in MS, it is advisable to rule out other causes first before assuming a new hearing problem is related to MS.

Taste and Smell

Disturbances of taste and smell are not common in MS. However, some studies suggest that problems in these areas occur more often in people with MS than in the general population, particularly in people with a more progressive disease course. There may be inability to taste or smell (**ageusia** and **anosmia**, respectively) or the presence of unpleasant tastes and odors (**dysgeusia** and **cacosmia**, respectively). Because these changes are so uncommon in MS, other causes should be investigated and ruled out before concluding that MS is the culprit.

Acute onset of problems with hearing, taste, or smell that are determined to be due to MS are usually treated in the same way as any exacerbation—with a short course of steroids.

Summary

Sensory symptoms are common in MS, particularly those related to pain and vision. While other sensory changes can occur, including problems with hearing, taste, or smell, they are more likely to be caused by conditions other than MS. It may be tempting to blame everything on your MS, but it is important for you and your health care providers to examine other possible causes for less common sensory symptoms to ensure no other health conditions are missed and that you get the appropriate treatment. Describe what you are experiencing to your MS care provider: what the sensations feel like; when and where they occur; what seems to trigger them; and what, if anything, helps them feel better. There is no reason to live with the kinds of discomfort that these sensory symptoms can cause.

CHAPTER 7

Mood and Cognition

In this chapter, you will learn:

- Common mood changes in multiple sclerosis
- Common changes in thinking and memory
- The impact of mood and cognition symptoms on each other and also on self-esteem, self-confidence, daily life, and relationships
- Assessment and treatment strategies

How Multiple Sclerosis Can Impact Mood

Feelings and moods are our constant companions. They impact how we view ourselves and others, as well as the world around us. Multiple sclerosis (MS) can affect mood in a variety of ways and for different reasons. Let's look at the most common changes and why they occur.

Grief

Grief is a strong, sometimes overwhelming feeling of loss, powerlessness, or even emptiness. It is a universal experience, but one that each person feels differently in relation to losses or changes in their life. Grief is constant (sometimes in the forefront and sometimes lurking in the background) for people whose lives are changed by symptoms that interfere with cherished abilities and roles, disrupt plans, and challenge relationships. Beginning with their diagnosis, people with MS have to give up the image they had of themselves before chronic illness came along and re-create a self-image that includes MS. This grieving process is a normal and natural response to unpredictable change and loss, and it will ebb and flow over the course of the disease. Although grieving can feel painful and, at times, overwhelming, it also allows for moments of laughter, joy, and connection with others. It is a healthy first step toward adaptation and problem-solving around whatever changes have occurred.

Depression

Depression is neither healthy nor normal. When someone with MS experiences ongoing feelings of sadness, despair, and hopelessness and/or a lack of enjoyment or pleasure in activities and relationships, along with heightened **irritability** or hypersensitivity, it's time to determine whether depression could be the cause. While these symptoms must occur all day, every day for at least 2 weeks to be diagnosed as a **major depression**, less severe forms of depression can also occur and can still feel overwhelming.

Feeling depressed makes everything else feel worse. People with MS who are depressed experience their other MS symptoms more intensely, including fatigue, pain, weakness, problems with thinking and memory, and sleep problems. Depression is very common in MS. Approximately half of people living with MS will experience a major depressive episode at some point in their disease; many more will experience milder, yet still debilitating, levels of depression. Depression is more than just a reaction to life with a chronic, unpredictable illness. It is also related to changes in the brain and immune system caused by the disease. In other words, depression is a symptom of MS, as worthy of careful diagnosis and management as any other symptom of the disease.

Anxiety

Anxiety can be described as intense, excessive, and persistent worry about everyday events or possible future events. Although we all feel worried or anxious at times about a specific situation or event, true anxiety can be overwhelming and overpowering. Like depression, intense anxiety is also very common in MS, and seems to be part of the disease itself, as well as a reaction to the unpredictability of the disease course. Wondering when the next "shoe will drop" is a common worry. Although anxiety in the face of a chronic, potentially disabling disease is normal, overwhelming anxiety that interferes with sleeping, daily activities, and relationships is not. As with depression, anxiety that feels crippling requires assessment and treatment.

Irritability

Irritability—feeling like a prickly pear—is a symptom reported by many with MS and confirmed by their support partners. While irritability can be a very common sign of depression, it can also stand on its own. It's uncomfortable for the person with MS, as well as for people around them. Along with irritability, many people with MS experience ups and downs in their moods that can be as confusing for them as they are for those around them. As with the other mood changes that can occur in MS, it's important to realize that relief is available.

The Importance of Early and Ongoing Screening

Mood changes impact quality of life, relationships, productivity, employment, and self-esteem. Because many people believe that mood changes are a sign of weakness, they may try to endure them, hide them, or self-medicate with alcohol or other substances. The fact is that these mood changes deserve attention from your health care team, just like your other symptoms. The current recommendation is for people with MS to be screened for depression at the time of diagnosis and every 6–12 months thereafter. Many would advocate for a similar screening for anxiety. If your primary care physician or MS care provider is not asking you about your mood on a routine basis, you can start by asking yourself the following two questions:

- During the past 2 weeks, have I often felt down, depressed, or hopeless?
- During the past 2 weeks, have I had little interest or pleasure in doing things?

If you answer "yes" to either or both of these questions, you may be experiencing depression. We encourage you to share this information with your provider so you can get the help you need. See Appendix 2 for free, confidential screenings offered by Mental Health America.

Treatment Options for Mood Changes

Managing mood is very personal. Some people lean toward talk therapy as a way to work through their feelings and get to a better place. Others shy away from talking and just want to take a pill. And still others want to use exercise or physical activity as a way to deal with their moods. The good news is that all three strategies can be helpful, and they may offer the best outcomes when used in combination.

Research has shown that talk therapy (particularly cognitive–behavioral therapy [CBT]) is effective for treating MS-related mood changes. CBT works by helping a person become aware of inaccurate, negative, or self-defeating thinking in order to view challenging situations more accurately and manage them more effectively. For some people, taking medication in addition to the talk therapy is necessary, particularly for those with severe depression and/or anxiety. Physical activity has also been shown to improve mood. A mental health professional can help you figure out the strategies that will work best for you. Several different types of mental health professionals are available.

Psychiatrists are physicians who specialize in the diagnosis and treatment of mental health issues. While some offer talk therapy as well, most diagnose mental health conditions and prescribe medication, if needed.

Psychologists specialize in the diagnosis and treatment of mental health problems, using primarily individual, family, and group therapy as treatment strategies. In some states, psychologists can also prescribe medication. **Health psychologists** specialize in the treatment of individuals living with chronic illness or disability.

Social workers and licensed professional counselors also diagnose mental health conditions and treat mental health problems with talk therapy.

One positive outcome of the COVID-19 pandemic has been the increased availability of virtual psychotherapy options. So even if you live in an area where mental health resources are limited, you are now more likely to be able to find a mental health professional who is licensed to offer services online.

As with all other aspects of MS care, effective management begins with you. Talk to your providers, self-advocate for screening and further assessment if needed, and seek treatment with a qualified mental health professional.

How Multiple Sclerosis Can Impact Cognition

Changes in thinking and memory (**cognitive dysfunction**) are very common in MS: At least 65% of people with MS experience cognitive challenges over the course of the disease. These changes can occur at any point in the disease—even as a first symptom—so it's important to know what they are and how to recognize them.

Slowed **information processing** is the hallmark of MS cognitive change. In everyday terms, this refers to the brain's inability to deal with incoming information as quickly and automatically as it used to. People find it difficult to keep up with conversations; respond as quickly or easily to questions; solve problems rapidly; or react to many stimuli at one time, such as when driving a car. The result is that people may feel that the world around them is simply moving too fast. When that happens, memory problems can also occur, simply because the person didn't hear or process something in the first place.

Memory problems are one of the cognitive difficulties people with MS report most often. Although memories from early life—such as the name of one's seventh-grade math teacher, the memory of one's first kiss, or the name of one's best friend in grade school—remain intact, activities that require **working memory** (e.g., remembering recent conversations, following the plot of a book or movie, traveling to a familiar place in one's neighborhood, remembering appointments, or remembering when to take medications) can become very challenging.

Attention and concentration are often impaired in MS. People who used to multitask as part of their everyday life may find they can no longer do so. "I'm lucky if I can get one thing done" is a common refrain. They are easily distracted from a task and then have trouble remembering what they were doing when they try to return to it. If there's noise in the background, following a conversation becomes very difficult, which makes it virtually impossible to remember that conversation later. For other people, their minds feel "sticky." They find it difficult to switch their focus from one task to another, even when they need to.

Word-finding problems, such as the "tip of the tongue" phenomenon, happen to all of us from time to time, but they are much more common in people with MS. They can interrupt the flow of conversations in ways that feel quite disruptive and embarrassing.

Problems with **visual–spatial processing**, or the ability to use visual information to correctly localize objects in space, can interfere with tasks such as following directions on a map, assembling a puzzle, or knowing which way to turn at a familiar intersection. These problems may also affect a person's ability to engage in sports activities or do-it-yourself projects.

Executive functions refer to the higher level cognitive tasks we do in our daily lives—for example, planning, solving problems, organizing, making decisions, using good judgment, and completing multistep tasks. Gradually, these complex processes may begin to feel difficult or impossible for someone with MS, impacting their ability to plan and organize home or work projects, pay bills, or strategize solutions for managing the unpredictable future.

In addition to these challenges, people with MS commonly report **cognitive fatigue**. Like physical fatigue, cognitive fatigue can come on suddenly, feel overwhelming, and stop you in your tracks. After working intensely for several minutes on a cognitive task, you may hit a wall, suddenly feeling unable to think or focus. In those moments, it's important to stop what you're doing, sit quietly and perhaps close your eyes, and give your brain a chance to rest. After this kind of break, you'll find yourself able to get back to work.

Effective Management Begins with Early and Ongoing Screening

Cognition experts currently recommend early and ongoing **cognitive screening** for people with MS to track changes in function. The simplest screening tool measures speed of information processing, which has been shown to be impacted at, or even before, the time of MS diagnosis. Early identification of cognitive challenges is important for several reasons:

- Cognitive problems, along with fatigue, are the most common reasons people with MS leave the workforce early.
- Problems with processing speed, attention, and memory impact conversations, relationships, and job performance.

- When a person's executive functions are impacted, they may have difficulty managing their household, planning their schedule, completing tasks such as paying bills or their income tax returns, attending appointments, or making sound decisions.

When Screening Is Positive, the Next Step Is an In-Depth Evaluation by a Cognition Specialist

When a **cognition specialist** (e.g., **neuropsychologist**, **speech–language pathologist**, or occupational therapist) performs testing on someone experiencing cognitive problems, their first step will be to assess the person's mood. Evaluating mood is important because, as discussed in this chapter, depression and anxiety, which are very common in people with MS, can impact cognition. So, treating mood symptoms may reduce many or all of the cognitive challenges someone with MS is experiencing.

An in-depth cognitive evaluation is helpful for many reasons. First, it helps establish a baseline from which changes in cognitive abilities can be measured over time. Tracking symptom progression is helpful for planning purposes, and in fact it becomes essential if, at any point, you need to apply for **Social Security disability (SSD)** benefits on the basis of cognitive difficulties. Second, in-depth testing also identifies your cognitive strengths along with the difficulties you are having. This will be helpful as you build tools and strategies to help compensate for difficulties and continue to complete everyday activities.

Cognitive evaluations vary in length and complexity. A standard evaluation can last from about 45 minutes to 4–6 hours. A full neuropsychological test battery (generally completed within several hours over 2 days), administered by a neuropsychologist, is required when applying for SSD. Under other circumstances, brief evaluations (45–60 minutes) conducted by a speech–language pathologist or occupational therapist can provide enough information about your cognitive strengths and challenges to make treatment recommendations.

Once Your Cognitive Evaluation Is Complete, Treatment Can Begin

A cognitive specialist can offer a range of cognitive exercises to improve your attention, memory, and other functions, and they can provide you with personalized compensatory tools and strategies for use in your daily activities. While performance on computerized exercises does tend to improve with practice, the benefits don't carry over very well to the real world, where there are many more distractions and complexities than in a therapy room. For this reason, developing strategies to compensate for cognitive difficulties has generally been found to be the more effective approach. While some neuropsychologists and psychologists offer cognitive remediation, the primary providers of these services are speech–language pathologists and occupational therapists, who may be easier to find in local communities.

Cognitive Remediation Evolves as Symptoms Evolve or Tasks Change

Regardless of the type of specialist you're working with, it's important to modify your compensatory tools and strategies as your needs change. You may, for example, work with a speech–language pathologist to develop strategies for managing tasks at home and work. After using those strategies for several months or years, you may find that new tools or strategies are needed. For example, a person who could at one time rely on their wall calendar to keep track of appointments may now need a smartwatch with alarms to give them frequent reminders. Or a person who used to be able to remember the steps involved in paying their bills may now need to use a task template that outlines the sequential steps (just like a recipe) for this multistep task. A re-evaluation of your cognitive functioning will help you and your remediation specialist update your toolbox to address your current challenges.

How Mood and Cognitive Changes Interact

By this point, we hope it's clear why mood and cognition are discussed together. They are intertwined in our brains, in our activities, and in our lives. A person who is very depressed or anxious is unable to think or reason effectively. Planning and problem-solving feel overwhelming. Decision-making is hampered by anxious thoughts and feelings of hopelessness or helplessness. And when people begin to experience cognitive changes that threaten their job performance and career, or challenge their ability to communicate effectively with family and friends, they may experience significant grief, as well as increased anxiety and/or depression. If you haven't been asked about your mood or cognition or haven't been screened for possible changes, it's time to advocate for yourself with your health care team. With early screening, you and your health care providers can identify any mood or cognitive changes that may be interfering with your daily activities and reducing your quality of life.

CHAPTER 8

Bladder and Bowel

In this chapter, you will learn:

- How multiple sclerosis can affect bladder and bowel
- Treatment and management strategies

Bladder and bowel issues include changes and challenges related to bladder and bowel function. While these types of symptoms are common in multiple sclerosis (MS), most can be effectively managed with lifestyle modifications and/or medications.

Normal Bladder Function

The bladder is like a big bag with a muscular wall. Its job is to stretch and fill with urine that comes from both kidneys. Normally, nerve receptors in the bladder can detect when about a cup of urine is present and can then send a "full" signal to the spinal cord. That signal travels to the brain, where it is interpreted and, if the place and timing are appropriate, an outgoing message is sent back to the bladder telling it to contract. At the same time, a message is given to the **sphincter muscle** (which controls the opening out of the bladder), allowing it to relax so that the urine can flow.

Both involuntary and voluntary activity are involved with healthy bladder function. For example, the signal that the bladder is full may be sent but you may not be able to go to a restroom at that moment, so your brain sends a voluntary signal to "hold" until the timing is better. In MS, several problems may arise that interfere with bladder function, categorized into three areas: difficulty holding urine in the bladder (urine storage), difficulty emptying the bladder, and a combined problem in which there is a disconnect between bladder contractions and sphincter activity.

Changes in Bladder Function

Bladder symptoms affect about three out of four people with MS. The most common symptoms of bladder dysfunction are urgency (gotta go!) and frequency (gotta go again . . . and again!). Other symptoms are also possible. Let's look at normal bladder function and issues that can arise in MS.

Difficulty with Urine Storage

Difficulty with urine storage, also called **detrusor–sphincter over-activity**, is the most common elimination problem in MS. This problem occurs when the bladder muscle (the **detrusor muscle**) is overactive and spastic. The signal that the bladder needs to be emptied occurs long before the bladder is full, which causes a person to feel a frequent need to urinate. The repeated signals produce abnormal bladder contractions that result in **urinary urgency**, **urinary frequency**, getting up multiple times during the night to urinate (**nocturia**), and sometimes urge **incontinence** (loss of bladder control due to urgency).

If you are experiencing this type of bladder issue, you know it can be very disruptive. When there are symptoms of urgency, you may experience significant fear of not having a restroom available when the urgent feeling strikes. You may feel tired from interrupted sleep. You may have some bladder leakage or dribbling. You may find yourself not wanting to leave the security of your home. If you are experiencing any of these challenges, it is definitely time for a conversation with your MS care provider. The following strategies that can help with a spastic and overactive bladder:

- Drink sufficient liquids to keep your urine a light straw color—usually about 1.5–2 liters per day.
- Drink about a cup of fluid every few hours. If you sip small amounts throughout the day, you're likely to experience more frequent urination and more sensations of urgency.
- Stop drinking fluids at least 2 hours before bedtime.
- Minimize or eliminate caffeinated beverages and alcoholic beverages as they provoke more urgency and frequency.
- If you smoke, seek assistance to stop. Among many other risks, smoking is a bladder irritant that causes more urgency.
- Ask your MS care provider about medications that can be considered for your symptoms.
- Talk to your MS provider about a referral to a urologist, especially one who specializes in neurologic causes of bladder problems.

A urologist may suggest bladder testing, known as **urodynamic testing**, which involves the following steps: First, a **urinary catheter** (thin tube) is inserted into the bladder. Fluid is then introduced into the bladder, after which measurements are made of pressures in the bladder (i.e., when the need to empty the bladder occurs, the amount of urine that is eliminated, and the amount of residual urine that remains in the bladder after urination). This testing identifies the bladder function problem that is occurring so that the correct treatment can be prescribed.

Percutaneous tibial nerve stimulation (PTNS) is a procedure in which a low electrical signal is used to stimulate the posterior tibial nerve (located on the inner ankle just above and behind the big inner ankle bone). This stimulation can reduce urgency and frequency in many people.

For persons who have not responded to medication or other measures, an implantable device that directly stimulates nerves to the bladder may also be helpful in treating overactive bladder symptoms. One drawback to this implantable device, however, is that it may limit the ability to undergo magnetic resonance imaging.

The urologist may also prescribe medications to reduce detrusor overactivity and relieve your symptoms, **pelvic floor physical therapy** to strengthen the muscles under the bladder and the tube that carries urine out of the body (the **urethra**), or other procedures if none of these resolve the problem.

Difficulty with Bladder Emptying

Sometimes the bladder fills and the signal to empty is disrupted somewhere along the spinal cord pathways. Symptoms may include urgency and frequency. You may also notice that your bladder does not feel empty after you urinate, which means you have emptied only some of the bladder's contents. Partial emptying can also cause frequent trips to the bathroom as well as loss of bladder control. Bladder infection may also occur when urine stays in the bladder too long.

Several strategies are available to help with this type of bladder problem. The first step is letting your MS provider know the symptoms you are experiencing, as they may refer you to a urologist for urodynamic testing (as described in the previous section) or for a procedure called **intermittent self-catheterization**. While very few individuals will be excited to consider self-catheterization, the procedure can be life-changing for those having bladder emptying issues. The procedure requires the introduction of a small tube (catheter) through the urethra and into the bladder to mechanically empty the bladder. Self-catheterizing may be done from one to several times a day based on individual need. This simple procedure can be done anywhere at any time—and gives you back the feelings of confidence and security you need to go about your daily activities.

Combined Dysfunction: Detrusor–Sphincter Dyssynergia

Multiple sclerosis can cause difficulty with functions involving the detrusor muscle and the sphincter. These functions become discoordinated, a problem called **detrusor–sphincter dyssynergia (DSD)**. DSD results in an overactive bladder muscle that cannot empty itself because the sphincter doesn't relax when it's supposed to. DSD produces symptoms of urgency, frequency, and incontinence, and it may also result in frequent bladder infections. Because DSD is a problem of both storage and emptying, treatment usually involves strategies to help calm down the overactive detrusor and simultaneously empty the bladder—for example, medication plus self-catheterization.

You may have noticed that the three types of bladder problems can produce similar symptoms: urgency, frequency, and occasional incontinence. For this reason, a careful evaluation by a urologist is important for ensuring that the right problem is being treated in the right ways.

Urinary Tract Infection

Urinary tract infections (UTIs) are common in the general population, particularly in women. And in MS, the risk and incidence are even greater. Urine is a sterile fluid, meaning very few or no bacteria are normally present. However, when urine becomes contaminated, a UTI can result. Most UTIs are treated easily with an oral antibiotic. However, an untreated and/or severe UTI can affect the kidneys, and in the worst case, it can affect the entire body, causing a life-threatening multisystem reaction to the infection known as **sepsis**.

UTIs have many causes. When a person is unable to empty their bladder completely and urine remains in the bladder for a long period of time, it can become contaminated with bacteria, potentially leading to a UTI. Bowel contaminants can also enter the bladder through the same tube (the urethra) from which urine exits the body. This is particularly common in women as the urethra is much shorter, and contaminants have easier access to the bladder, where the infection initially takes place.

Other factors that can contribute to UTIs include sexual inter-course, conditions that block the urinary tract (e.g., kidney stones), non-MS conditions that make it difficult to fully empty the bladder (e.g., an enlarged prostate in men), diabetes, urinary catheters, and not drinking enough fluids.

Symptoms of a UTI include burning pain with urination, lower abdominal or pelvic pain, increased urgency and frequency, voiding very small amounts, blood in the urine, strong odor to the urine, fever and chills, nausea, and fatigue. If you have MS, these symptoms can certainly be present with a UTI, but UTI symptoms may also present much differently. For example, common UTI symptoms such as pain or burning with urination may not be ap-parent in people with MS, and if there is already urgency and fre-quency as a result of MS, these symptoms may not seem much different with a UTI.

The potential impact of a UTI can be significant. If you have had other MS symptoms in the past or are living with current symptoms, a UTI can temporarily make those symptoms feel worse. While this is considered a pseudo-relapse and not an actual relapse (see Chapter 3 for more on relapses), it can still be extremely un-comfortable. Common MS symptoms that worsen with a UTI may include fatigue, cognitive problems, weakness, and stiffness or spas-ticity in the legs.

For some, these MS-related symptoms may be the first or only clue that a UTI is present. And whether the symptoms are the typical UTI symptoms or not so typical, a call to your primary care physician (PCP) or MS care provider is important so that appropriate treatment can be initiated. UTIs are treatable!

Treating a UTI

A urine sample will be needed to establish the presence of an infection and identify the bacterial culprit, and then an antibiotic will likely be prescribed. Should UTIs become a recurring problem (more than two per year), your PCP or MS care provider will likely refer you to a urologist, who will do a more comprehensive assessment to determine the best treatment plan.

Reducing Your Risk of Getting a UTI

In addition to seeking treatment for a UTI, there are also things you can do to reduce your risk of getting a UTI. These actions are not treatment for an active infection but can help you avoid developing a UTI. After sexual intercourse, try to empty your bladder and then wipe (front to back for women) with a warm washcloth or wet wipe; drink plenty of fluids to keep the urine a light straw color; try daily cranberry tablets (the juice does not work as well), which can help keep bacteria from sticking to the bladder wall; do your best to keep the pelvic area clean and dry; and try to keep the bowels moving regularly (see the next section on bowel symptoms) as a full bowel makes it difficult to empty the bladder completely.

Bowel Symptoms

More than 50% of people with MS report issues with bowel function.

Normal Bowel Function

Under normal circumstances, there is constant communication between the bowel and the brain, with signals of "full" being sent to the brain and signals to "go" or "not go" being sent back down to the bowel. Inner and outer sphincter muscles, as well as the pelvic floor muscles, must relax, allowing the muscles in the colon to push the stool out of the bowel. As with urinary function, there are involuntary and voluntary components to bowel function. MS can disrupt signals along the communication pathways between the brain and bowel; these disruptions may result in constipation, bowel leakage, or both. These problems can be frustrating as well as embarrassing, causing many people with these symptoms to avoid leaving the house or socializing with others.

Constipation

Constipation can result from disruption of nerve signals. It can also result from other factors, including decreased overall physical mobility, a diet low in fiber content, insufficient fluid intake, depressed mood, and side effects from medications. Useful strategies to relieve constipation include

- drinking plenty of noncaffeinated fluids;
- eating foods rich in fiber, such as fruits, vegetables, whole grains, and nuts;
- choosing a regular time to attempt a bowel movement every day;
- drinking a warm liquid, even warm water, before attempting a bowel movement; and
- increasing physical activity; if this is a challenge due to physical symptoms of MS, a referral to physical therapy may be helpful.

Sometimes, additional help with a stool softener or suppository is needed to facilitate bowel movements about three or four times a week. Laxatives or enemas may be used occasionally, but their use should always be discussed with your medical or MS provider beforehand. There are many types of laxatives on the market, with some being much more irritating for the bowel than others. Your provider can point you to the safest and least irritating options, although these medications should only be used occasionally regardless of their potential for irritation, as their continued use can lead to dependence. Because of this, your optimal strategy for managing constipation begins with dietary changes.

Bowel Incontinence

Fewer people with MS have episodes of bowel incontinence than with constipation. However, incontinence can occur with MS for a few reasons. For example, a person with reduced sensation in the rectum may be caught by surprise by a bowel movement. Or stool may move suddenly and quickly through the bowel and be expelled before they can get to the bathroom. Or a person with constipation may experience incontinence when loose stool from higher in the bowel leaks around hardened stool that is lodged in the colon or rectum. Whether the amount is large or small, the experience of bowel incontinence is embarrassing and upsetting. The fear of bowel incontinence is enough to make many people avoid all social activities. However, this is a problem that can be successfully treated for the vast majority of people who experience it. Treatments may include

- assessment of and changes to diet to ensure it is balanced with sufficient fiber;
- elimination of laxative or enema overuse;
- treatment of constipation; and
- medications that may help slow down bowel motility.

A comprehensive bowel program can help you establish an optimal diet for your bowel, a schedule for regular elimination, and an exercise regimen to help maintain healthy bowel function. If there is concern that a non-MS problem is the cause of the symptoms or the above treatments are ineffective, a referral to a gastroenterologist may need to be considered.

Bladder and Bowel Function Impact One Another and Can Also Impact Other Multiple Sclerosis Symptoms

The first thing many people do when they begin to experience bladder issues is to cut back on their liquid intake. However, taking in sufficient liquids is essential for both healthy bladder and bowel function. Because of this, if you are experiencing problems with both bladder and bowel function due to MS, your best strategy may be to tackle your bladder issues first so that you can drink adequate fluids without having to worry about urgency, frequency, or incontinence. Once your bladder is functioning more predictably, you may find that your constipation is improving because you are drinking more. But if not, you can focus on increasing your fluids, fiber, and exercise to get constipation under control.

When the bladder or bowel is consistently full and urination and/or bowel movements are incomplete, other MS symptoms may be aggravated. Lower extremity stiffness or spasticity can feel worse with a full bowel or bladder. Pain symptoms may also feel worse. When the bowel is full, many people feel sluggish or more fatigued.

Summary

Bladder symptoms (problems with emptying or storing urine or a combination of the two) and bowel symptoms (most often constipation) are quite common in MS. If you are experiencing these types of symptoms, you may feel that they are not related to your MS or that your MS care provider does not have the time to discuss these issues in a short follow-up appointment. But these symptoms can disrupt your life and prevent you from participating in the activities you enjoy. A thorough assessment and/or referral to the appropriate specialist can lead to effective treatment—and get you back to the fun activities you've been missing.

Section 3

Health and Wellness

CHAPTER 9

Your Overall Health and Wellness

In this chapter, you will learn:

- What comorbidities are—and why they matter
- Strategies for taking control of your health and well-being

If you have a recent diagnosis of multiple sclerosis (MS), you have a lot on your mind and may not be thinking about your overall health and wellness Or, if you have had MS for some time, your energy and focus may be on challenges you are experiencing with your MS, leaving little time or headspace to consider anything else. However, attending to overall health and well-being is important for everyone, and has significant implications for people with MS.

Comorbidity

A comorbidity or comorbid health condition is an additional condition or disease that a person has along with another condition (e.g., MS), which is not a complication of the first condition. Examples include diabetes or cancer in someone with MS, or high blood pressure in someone with psoriasis or lupus. Over the past decade, a lot of research has been done to better understand comorbidities in people with MS—which ones are most common and what effect they have on the course of someone's MS, adherence to disease-modifying therapies (DMTs), and overall quality of life.

The research has shown that certain comorbid conditions are more common in people with MS. An extensive review published in 2015 showed the following to be the most common comorbidities in people with MS:

- Depression
- Anxiety
- Hypertension
- Hypercholesterolemia (high cholesterol)
- Chronic lung disease

We also know that the **vascular comorbidities**—hypertension, high cholesterol, and ischemic heart disease—are more prevalent in people with MS than in the general population. Multiple research studies have confirmed the increased risk of cardiovascular disease in people with MS. Other conditions that are more prevalent in people with MS include migraine, chronic lung disease, and sleep disorders. Depression and anxiety have been identified as comorbid conditions in people with MS but are also known to be symptoms of MS (see Chapter 7). Given that mood changes can occur for a variety of reasons (symptom of MS, reaction to the challenges of a chronic illness, genetic predisposition, among others), it may not be possible to determine precisely the cause(s). Research on the risk of cancer in people with MS has yielded conflicting results, with some studies indicating a greater risk, whereas others do not.

Evidence is growing that obesity can contribute to vascular comorbidities such as heart disease, hypertension, and diabetes. In addition, there are indications from recent studies that obesity may also worsen neurologic outcomes.

Why Does This Matter?

Most people, whether they have MS or not, develop a range of health conditions as they get older. What does this mean for you if you have MS?

- Vascular comorbidities and chronic lung disease, as well as depression, have been found to be associated with increased MS disability progression.
- The presence of comorbidities at the onset of MS can make getting an accurate and timely MS diagnosis more challenging because there are so many factors at play at the same time.
- Having multiple comorbidities at the time of diagnosis is also associated with greater disability progression.
- Some comorbid conditions make it impossible to use certain MS DMTs.
- Comorbidities can also contribute to earlier mortality.

We know that none of that was easy to read. But the positive news is that many of the comorbid conditions that are more prevalent in MS can be prevented or modified with lifestyle behaviors and preventive health. Our goal is to point you toward strategies that can help you optimize your overall health and reduce the potential impact of co-morbid health conditions on your MS.

Taking Control of Your Health and Wellness

Let's look at the behaviors that can help you stay as healthy and as comorbidity-free as possible.

Stopping Smoking

Stopping smoking is never easy. But it's something you may want to consider in order to reduce your risk for vascular and lung disease and improve your health. In addition to comorbidity risks associated with smoking, smoking and second-hand smoke are known to increase physical disability in MS.

Staying Active

Staying active is beneficial and does not have to mean sweating it out at the gym. Any and all activities you participate in throughout the day are helpful for improving your strength, flexibility, balance, cardiovascular health, mood, and cognitive functioning—and increasing these activities is even more helpful. For many people with physical disability from their MS, increasing their amount of physical activity is challenging. A physical therapist or exercise specialist with expertise in MS can assess your abilities and help you design activities that work for you. See Chapter 11 for more specific information about exercise and physical activity.

Optimizing Your Diet

The foods you eat can impact your risk of vascular comorbidities and your overall health (see Chapter 12). The Mediterranean diet has been shown to reduce the risk of vascular comorbidities in the general population. Data from several small but controlled trials of the Mediterranean diet in persons with MS suggest that it may improve function and some symptoms, although larger trials are needed to confirm benefit. As no specific diet has been found through controlled research to change the course of MS, the following are general dietary recommendations for good health:

- Plan your meals ahead and prepare them at home.
- Make sure that at least half of your plate contains colorful fresh fruits and vegetables.

- If you choose to eat grains, choose whole grains over refined grains.
- Avoid processed foods and sugars as much as you can.
- Adequate fluid and fiber intake is essential for the health of your bowel and bladder. (See Chapter 8 on bladder and bowel.)

Attending to Mood Changes

Regular screening for depression or other mood disorders by your MS provider or primary care physician (PCP) can identify mental health issues that may require further evaluation and treatment (see Chapter 7 for more information about mood changes in MS and current screening recommendations).

Managing Stress

Stress can be both positive and negative. When positive, stress prompts us to immediate action—typically away from an immediate or anticipated threat to our physical safety. Stress can also be a complex physical and/or emotional response to an event, a workplace issue, finances, or illness. In these cases, it can act as a signal that we need to take constructive action to address the situation.

Stress can be experienced over a brief period of time (acute) or a long period of time (chronic), such as with an illness like MS. Particularly when it's chronic, stress can have negative health effects—such as elevation in blood pressure, heart attack, heart disease, headaches, indigestion, poor sleep, erectile dysfunction, decreased libido, difficulties with concentration, and weight gain. Stress can also make decision-making and problem-solving more difficult, provoke anger, and challenge relationships.

Often, our attempts to manage stress on our own take the form of unhealthy behaviors such as overeating, smoking, and/or increased alcohol or drug intake. Recognizing that stress exists and identifying the stressor or stressors are key steps in managing and reducing the stress—and shifting from unhealthy to healthy behaviors to manage it.

For people with MS, having a chronic illness that is unpredictable may feel overwhelming. Challenges with low energy, cognitive challenges, bladder issues, walking difficulties, and other symptoms are stressful. Reducing stress does not happen overnight, but stress-lowering activities include the following:

- Talking to your MS care provider about symptoms or other issues that feel overwhelming and stressful
- Considering requests for help—which may initially feel embarrassing—can help relieve your stress in the long term
- Doing something you enjoy each day, such as reading, walking, gardening, watching a movie, or listening to a podcast
- Connecting with your support system
- Trying for regular physical activity within the limits of your abilities and challenges
- Trying a mindfulness activity (See Appendix 2 for information about mindfulness and resources to get you started.)

Attending to Preventive Health Screening

Talk with your PCP about the recommended screening schedule for various comorbid conditions, such as cancers, high blood pressure, high cholesterol, cardiac conditions, diabetes, and depression. Your PCP will monitor your weight, help with smoking cessation, treat infections, recommend immunizations, and treat other conditions. For women, regular women's health (gynecology) visits will assess your overall health and screen for infections, abnormalities of reproductive organs, and cancers. Additional preventive health measures include regular dental check-ups (which can identify hidden infections in your gums that can trigger inflammatory activity); vision exams; and, for many, regular skin checks for skin cancer or other abnormalities.

Staying Current with Immunizations

Immunizations help prevent many types of infections (mostly those caused by viruses) or lessen the risk of serious illness from an infection. For people with MS, infections can stimulate the immune system and worsen MS symptoms. And an infection-related fever can provoke a pseudo-exacerbation (see Chapter 1). In addition, if mobility is compromised, you may be more prone to certain bacterial infections such as pneumonia, urinary tract infections, or skin breakdown related to a pressure sore.

MS DMTs affect the immune system, and some of them may impact the safety and/or effectiveness of immunizations. Talking about immunizations with your MS provider can help you understand the risks and benefits of vaccines and inform your decision-making.

Getting Restorative Sleep

The appropriate amount of restful sleep will help you feel and function at your best. Poor sleep can exacerbate your MS fatigue and may contribute to other MS symptoms, such as cognitive problems or depression. Contributors to poor sleep in people with MS include the following:

- Spasticity or nighttime spasms in the muscles
- Needing to empty the bladder during the night
- Napping during the day
- Medications such as corticosteroids or stimulants to help with daytime sleepiness
- Limited physical activity
- Depression and other mood problems
- Pain, which often feels worse at night
- Sleep disorders that are more common in MS, such as restless legs

Here are a few tips to help with your sleep:

- Choose a consistent time to go to bed and get up every day, including weekends.
- Make your bed the place for sleep and sex only.
- Avoid TV and electronics, at bedtime which may disrupt your ability to fall asleep.
- Avoid drinking fluids at least 2 hours before bed to minimize nighttime trips to the bathroom.
- Limit any caffeine to the morning hours.
- Limit alcohol use.
- Create an evening activity routine that winds down an hour or so before bed.
- Consider using calming music or meditation prior to trying to sleep.
- If you do not fall asleep within 15–20 minutes, get up. Watch a little TV, listen to music, or read for a little while—then return to bed and try to fall asleep.

Restorative sleep is vital for general good health as well as having an impact on other MS problems. If you are having difficulty falling asleep or staying asleep, let your PCP or MS care provider know about it so that you can explore the possible causes and collaboratively identify solutions.

Summary

When living with MS, attending to your overall health can enhance your daily life and well-being. Comorbid conditions can delay an accurate MS diagnosis and lead to greater MS disability. Many comorbid conditions are preventable or modifiable through lifestyle behaviors. Attention to activity, diet, stress, overall mood, and sleep contributes to overall health and wellness. In addition, regular visits with a PCP, dentist, ophthalmologist, dermatologist, and, for women, an obstetrician/gynecologist can help screen for comorbid conditions and offer early intervention should a problem be identified.

CHAPTER 10

Care Partners, Support Partners, Carers, and Caregivers

This Is About You

In this chapter, you will learn:

- What it means to be a **care partner**
- Why multiple sclerosis has been called a "we disease" rather than a "me disease"
- How to live more comfortably with the unpredictability of multiple sclerosis
- How to navigate the invisible symptoms of multiple sclerosis symptoms
- Ways to maintain a full and active life
- How to work effectively with your partner's health care team
- Why caring for yourself is so important

You may be a partner or spouse, parent, other family member, or friend, and you may be providing a substantial amount of hands-on help, emotional support, or other types of assistance. Whatever your specific role is currently, learning how to care for yourself while caring for someone else is important.

We use the term *care partner* or *support partner* to describe anyone who provides help and support to a person with multiple sclerosis (MS). This term makes it clear that care and support work best when there's a true partnership. Ideally, we are always support partners for each other in our important relationships, with each person giving and receiving and each person feeling like a valued member in the relationship. However, when one person lives with a chronic, unpredictable illness, the balance in the partnership may shift periodically or over time. During a relapse, or if the person with MS experiences increased disability, the person providing the support may have to take on a more active, hands-on role. When this occurs, we refer to them as **caregivers**. Yet even when MS is quite disabling, there are ways for partners to continue to support one another and attend to each other's wellness.

In the medical literature, those who provide care to someone who is ill or disabled have been called "the invisible patients." And there's a good reason for this: Care partners, particularly those who provide extensive, hands-on care for someone else, are known to have health challenges of their own, higher rates of depression and anxiety, and overwhelming fatigue. Family, friends, and the health care community are so focused on the health and needs of the "patient" that the well-being of the support person is overlooked. Many are seldom or never asked how they are doing. And the support partner may feel selfish or guilt-ridden for having feelings and needs of their own when they're the "healthy one."

So, what does this mean for support partner wellness and self-care? Let's look at some common challenges that support partners face and the strategies that can help manage them:

Acknowledging Feelings and Fears

It is rare for people who say "till death do us part" or "besties forever" to know what lies in the future. We don't anticipate severe illness or disability or major changes in our roles and relationships, but they happen: It is natural and normal to have feelings when things change. When life changes, dreams for the future are disrupted, a partnership is altered by physical or cognitive changes, or daily life becomes dictated by the demands of MS, we feel grief. We also feel anxiety over the "what-ifs" associated with an unpredictable illness.

Stephen has been married to Joan for 25 years, and for 20 of those years, Joan has had MS. Over the past 5 years or so, her symptoms have progressed significantly, affecting both her mobility and her cognitive abilities—leading to her recent retirement on disability from her job as a teacher. She has difficulty managing her daily activities and needs help with most household tasks and self-care activities.

Stephen finds himself overwhelmed by his increased responsibilities, including all the cooking and cleaning, errands, taking Joan to doctor appointments, and handling the increasing paperwork associated with Joan's insurance claims. On top of his demanding job, these responsibilities leave him feeling drained and exhausted. His sleep is disturbed by having to help Joan to the bathroom multiple times and by his own worries about their finances, their ability to remain in their home, the progression of Joan's MS, and what would happen if he were to become ill or disabled. Ensuring that Joan has the loving care she needs remains his top priority. Most painful of all is Stephen's loneliness. He misses his vibrant, lively, and engaging partner; their partnership has changed in ways he had never anticipated.

Lurking in the back of his mind is a growing feeling of resentment at how much their lives have changed and how little time he now has for himself. His own social, recreational, and wellness activities have all gone by the wayside as his support partner role has evolved.

Resentment and anger over things changing, sacrifices that must sometimes be made, and feeling out of control are normal, as is guilt over feelings and thoughts that may not feel "nice" or align with personal values. You're not alone if you find yourself thinking "I wish it would just go away," "I don't know how long I can do this," or "This isn't what I signed up for." Acknowledging your feelings is the first step to figuring out how to manage and deal with them. And as you begin to explore those feelings, your next step is to figure out which of them you feel you can deal with on your own or with your loved one, which ones you might want to talk over with a close friend or in a support group, and which ones you might want to talk over more privately with a mental health professional. Reaching out for support is a sign of strength and emotional resilience, not weakness. It gives you the opportunity to learn more about yourself, examine your feelings without judgment, and figure out how to live more comfortably with them.

If your feelings begin to feel overwhelming, you're not alone. Depression and anxiety are common in care partners for those with chronic illness and disability. Because others are unlikely to ask you how you're doing or feeling, it rests with you to seek help and support from your own health care provider if your emotions feel too hot or painful to handle. A counselor or therapist with expertise in chronic illness and disability can help you identify and manage your feelings, find ways to talk about them in respectful and productive ways, and help you feel supported and less alone.

But if you ever find yourself saying or doing things that you wouldn't want others to hear or see, that could be a clear sign that you're feeling overwhelmed and at your limit. This doesn't make you a bad person—but it does mean that you could use more help and support than you're currently receiving.

Ellie and Frank have been married for 17 years and living with MS for 10 years. Recently, Frank's needs for assistance have increased significantly, and he becomes very anxious when

Ellie isn't around. Ellie has been feeling trapped between the demands of her job; Frank's needs, which feel constant; and the needs of their two teenage children. Lately, she's found herself acting "not like herself" at home and at work She loses her temper a lot—with Frank, the kids, and her colleagues; has been much less gentle than she used to be while assisting Frank; and has said some very hurtful things that she wishes she could take back. And because of her very demanding schedule, Ellie hasn't been able to spend time with her women friends, who have always added joy, humor, and comfort to her life. Ellie is reaching her physical and emotional limits and needs help and support.

If you're noticing these kinds of changes in yourself, multiple resources are available (see Appendix 2), including MS **advocacy organizations**, caregiver organizations, mental health professionals, or your own health care provider(s). They can offer you information, emotional support, and referrals to mental health professionals and caregiver organizations. Taking that first step is the most difficult, but the relief you'll feel will be your reward.

Getting a Handle on the Unpredictability of Multiple Sclerosis

It is important to remember that no two people have MS in exactly the same way and the symptoms can vary, even over the course of a day. No one can predict the future for a person with MS, and although planning for an unpredictable future is challenging, it is the best way to create a safety net. Think together with your partner how you can make yourselves feel more secure and less vulnerable if things change. A few things to consider, at the outset, include the following:

- Finding an expert financial planner who specializes in helping those with a disability
- Identifying housing/neighborhood options in the event your current living situation becomes unmanageable, and joining a waiting list
- Considering career options if a change becomes necessary
- Getting life and disability insurance for yourself

No one makes the best decisions in a crisis; some preplanning can relieve worry and help you feel more prepared. In other words, you want to plan for the worst while hoping for the best. In most instances, the worst "what-ifs" you worry about don't happen. So, this isn't about being pessimistic or hopeless; rather, it's about giving yourselves the best safety net possible.

Learning How to Navigate the Invisible Symptoms of Multiple Sclerosis

In previous chapters, we shared insight and guidance about what a person living with MS might expect. But as a support partner, you may often find it difficult to know what your loved one is experiencing physically or emotionally, or how their cognitive abilities may be changing. Fatigue, problems with thinking and memory, pain, and emotional changes such as anxiety and depression are common symptoms of MS. There may be days when your partner with MS looks fine but is feeling drained, weak, extremely uncomfortable, or distracted, forgetful, and disorganized. If they don't tell you, you probably have little idea what's actually going on. This is frustrating for them, and it is frustrating and mystifying for you. You may wonder when to help and when to step back, particularly if your partner gives you mixed signals—resentful one moment that you're not helping enough and then resentful the next moment for helping too much, hovering, or being too protective.

> *Larry and Janet are living with Janet's relapsing MS. Janet wants to be as independent as possible when she feels well but needs assistance from Larry when her symptoms are acting up. Larry is struggling to know when and how to help and support Janet, but he is feeling frustrated and confused by Janet's confusing messages:*
>
> *Monday morning: "I feel fine—please stop hovering and treating me like a . . . sick person . . . child. I want to do things myself!"*
> *Later that same day: "Can't you see how awful I feel? If you . . . loved me . . . paid any attention . . . understood my MS, you'd be more helpful."*
> *Larry feels as though he's walking on eggshells, never quite doing the right things at the right time even though he's trying his best to be responsive.*

Finding a way to communicate in the moment about symptoms and needs can help eliminate guesswork for the support partner. A person with MS who shares hand signals, little signs or notes (thumbs up/down, green light/red light, gas tank full or empty, or "I'm fine now"/"I need help now") can help their support partner understand the frequent ups and downs of MS without having to explain it all the time. No support partner, no matter how loving they are, can read their partner's mind, so consider having a conversation with your partner about what kind of signaling system might work for the two of you. If conflicting needs and concerns continue to interfere with your relationship, a good counselor or therapist can help you learn more effective ways to communicate with one another.

Maintaining a Full and Interesting Life When Multiple Sclerosis Seems to Get in the Way

Many couples living with MS start to feel that their world is shrinking, with fewer activities, a waning social life, less travel, and fewer windows of time for engaging in individual or shared activities.

Staying Active Together

The best strategy for staying active together with activities you enjoy is to consider doing your favorite activities differently and/or exploring new activities. Thinking about doing things differently isn't easy, because no one likes to give up activities or hobbies they enjoy. But assistive devices and mobility aids—when they're needed—can open up a lot of doors. A tool-chest of devices allows the whole family to share in enjoyable activities together. In other words, the whole family benefits from these devices, not just the person with MS.

Staying Connected with Friends and Family

Many support partners find that some friends and extended family begin to shy away or even disappear. This can happen for a variety of reasons. Perhaps they don't know what to say or do in relation to the MS, so they awkwardly back off. Others get frustrated with last-minute changes of plans, and others can't offer the accessibility the person with MS needs. Some friends simply stop asking after their invitations have been turned down several times.

The best way to maintain or regain your social life is to take steps to help others feel more comfortable: Invite them to your house for pizza or suggest an accessible restaurant; suggest an activity that everyone can share; ask if they have any questions about MS that you can answer; let people know you miss seeing them. And always have a plan B for any social engagement so you can change course and do something simpler, such as takeout at your house.

Staying Active Yourself

It is important to keep in mind that you and your partner don't always have to do everything together. Have a conversation about shared activities you enjoy as well as individual activities you want to make time for. Taking time for your own hobbies, physical activities, and friends is important for your own wellness. While you may not be able to do as many of those things as you did before, make sure you carve out at least a little time each week for the activities that sustain you. If you need a friend or neighbor to stay with your partner while you're out, ask them for a time that might work for them—and offer to bring back a pizza for their family dinner or help them in some other way.

Gaining Recognition from and Connection with the Multiple Sclerosis Care Team

As a partner, spouse, or family member of a person with MS, you have a key role to play with the health care team. Although the person with MS is the primary focus of the team's care, your input matters. With the permission of the person with MS, it is extremely helpful for you to be present during medical appointments for several reasons:

- You provide an extra pair of ears, perhaps even taking notes, to help the person with MS remember all that was said.
- Your input about how things have been going since the last visit is helpful to the providers.
- You are able to convey what's reasonable or not about the treatment plan, including your degree of availability to assist with medications, toileting, exercises, or other hands-on tasks.

- The health care team is more likely to take your health and well-being into account when the team can see and hear from you.

Making Your Own Health and Wellness a Priority

Taking care of yourself isn't selfish; rather, it's self-sustaining and essential. It's only when you are your own best self that you can help another person. The following are suggestions for self-care:

- Take time for your own medical and dental check-ups.
- Stay up to date with your immunizations.
- Carve out time in your week for the recommended 150 minutes of exercise and/or physical activity and exercise.
- Try to get the amount of sleep you need, adjusting your bedtime, finding time for a nap, or doing whatever else you have to do to get a good rest.
- Pay attention to your own moods and feelings.
- Create a support network that gives you emotional support, assistance with tasks, company for the person with MS so you can get some time to yourself, and a social outlet.
- If you feel overwhelmed, exhausted, or totally stressed out— reach out.

Summary

Being a support partner can make you feel proud, physically exhausted, emotionally overwhelmed, closer than ever to your partner, or lonesome for the partnership that's been changed by MS. It is a challenging role that you don't need to handle all on your own. Engage with the MS care team as much as you can (or as your partner permits). The MS advocacy organizations are there to support you and help you find the resources and support you need.

CHAPTER 11

Exercise and Physical Activity

In this chapter, you will learn:

- The benefits of an active lifestyle for physical, emotional, cognitive, and social well-being
- The recommended amount of physical activity and exercise for people with multiple sclerosis
- Ways to remain active through structured exercise and physical activities
- How you and your partner can remain active together despite multiple sclerosis

Why Staying Active Is So Important

"Exercise is medicine" is a relatively new way of thinking in the health care realm. Researchers throughout the world have been conducting studies to demonstrate the impact of physical activity and exercise on many aspects of our health, including brain plasticity (the ability of the nervous system to rewire its activity in response to growth, change, and damage), physical health, mood, cognitive functions (see Chapter 9), and the **gut microbiota**. The growing body of research suggests that exercise and physical activity provide many benefits over our lifetime. Today, many health care providers, including those providing multiple sclerosis (MS) care, routinely promote exercise as part of their treatment recommendations.

The Benefits of Physical Activity and Exercise for People with Multiple Sclerosis

Researchers have demonstrated that exercise is safe for people with MS and that it provides additional benefits for immune function and quality of life. We've known for some time that exercise can help with MS symptom management: improving strength, balance, and coordination and reducing fatigue, constipations, and stiffness or spasticity. But in addition to those benefits, it is now know that exercise has some impact on disease activity and progression, as well as on disease prevention.

> *Angela, a 35-year-old married woman, has recently been diagnosed with MS. Her MS provider sees in her electronic medical record that she is also being treated for high blood pressure, type 1 diabetes, and periodic episodes of depression. The provider talks with Angela about starting a disease-modifying therapy as soon as possible but also emphasizes how important it is for her to continue managing the comorbid conditions she has along with her MS. He lets her know that comorbid conditions, particularly vascular ones such as diabetes and high blood pressure, have been shown to speed the progression of MS and contribute to a shortened life span. And depression, which can be a symptom of MS as well as a reaction to its challenges, can make it more difficult for her to engage in the wellness activities that are important to her overall health.*
>
> *Angela's provider explains that exercise and physical activity will not only help her manage her comorbidities but also reduce her fatigue and improve her mood. He refers her to a physical therapist (PT) for an assessment and recommendations on how she can engage in more exercise and physical activity despite the MS fatigue and bouts of weakness she is experiencing.*

Research has shown that by the time of their diagnosis, people with MS already have more comorbid health conditions, including depression and vascular conditions (see Chapter 9), than people in the general population. Exercise and physical activity can help prevent and reduce these conditions, which in turn benefits MS. Hence the emphasis on exercise as medicine in MS care.

And yet, people with MS are much less active than their non-MS counterparts in the general population for a variety of reasons, including fatigue and other MS symptoms, safety concerns, environmental barriers, limited support from family or their health care provider, and lack of self-confidence. So, let's discuss the current recommendations for people with MS and some strategies you can use to maintain or increase your physical activity level.

Exercise and Physical Activity Recommendations for Adults with Multiple Sclerosis

The current recommendation from the National Multiple Sclerosis Society, based on input from clinical and research experts in MS, rehabilitation, and physical activity, is at least 150 minutes of exercise and/or 150 minutes of lifestyle physical activity per week. Physical activity encompasses any bodily movement that results from muscle contractions and increases a person's expenditure of energy. It encompasses **lifestyle physical activities**, which include any occupational, household, or leisure activity that requires energy expenditure, such as dressing and grooming, cleaning, cooking, walking the dog, dancing, making a bed, or cutting the grass, as well as **structured exercise**, which is performed repeatedly over time with a specific goal (e.g., exercise training to improve strength, endurance, balance, and flexibility). All activity counts toward your 150 minutes per week.

Structured exercise and lifestyle physical activity are distinct from rehabilitation (also provided by PTs and occupational therapists [OTs]), which uses targeted strategies to help you regain or maintain physical function (e.g., following an MS relapse) and promote safety and independence (see Chapter 3).

While You May Think You Can't, You Actually Can

People with MS may have many varied reactions to the recommendation for more exercise and physical activity.

"I Worry About Making My MS Worse or Injuring Myself"

Years of research has shown that exercise is safe for people with MS. It will not cause you harm or make the disease worse. Physical activity offers you many benefits for both your MS and your overall health and well-being. Before you start any new physical activity or exercise, talk about it with your MS provider The members of your health care team can recommend activities that are safe for you, regardless of your ability level, and recommend aids or tools to help you do them comfortably. They will help you reduce your fall risk, increase your energy, improve your sleep, reduce constipation, and help you be more independent in your everyday activities. There is a lot to be gained. You can feel better, healthier, stronger, more confident, and safer.

"I Don't Have the Energy to Exercise—I'm Just Too Tired All the Time"

Physical activity and exercise geared to your abilities comprise one of the best strategies for reducing your fatigue and building your endurance. The key is to start slowly and build gradually. Pay attention to how your body feels, stop when you need to rest, and be patient with yourself as you gradually add to your activities.

"When I Try to Exercise, I Feel Worse Afterward Than I Did Before"

Listening to your body is important. Many people try to do too much too fast or for too long, and then they pay for it for the next couple of days. Pace yourself and stop before you hit a wall. Start with just a few minutes of activity and increase it as you feel able. Over time, your endurance will increase. And if you're sensitive to heat and humidity, as many people with MS are, you may find that your symptoms temporarily worsen when you exercise, just as they do when you have a fever or stay outdoors in the heat. This temporary flare-up of symptoms (referred to as a pseudoexacerbation) causes no additional nerve damage and will subside when your body cools down. You can help your body remain cool by wearing a cooling vest, bandanna, hat, or wristbands and drinking cold water while you exercise.

"Everything Takes Me So Long Now; I Just Don't Have Time"

Fitting physical activity into your day isn't as difficult as you think—especially if you decide to make it a self-care priority. First, remember that all of your regular daily activities count toward your total weekly goal of 150 minutes of exercise. Getting showered and dressed, making the bed, washing dishes, mowing the lawn, folding laundry, and shopping for groceries are examples of built-in mini workouts in everyday life. Second, you don't have to get your daily exercise all at once. Whether you do 30 minutes all at one time or do 1- to 3-minute bits throughout the day, the benefits are the same. See Appendix 2 for information about how to sprinkle exercise over the course of your day.

"If I Can't Do My Favorite Activities the Way I Used to, I'm Just Not Interested"

In some ways, this is the toughest barrier to overcome because it requires you to grieve over the losses you have experienced and allow yourself to think about new possibilities. The grieving is the hard part, but the new possibilities are endless. Many of your favorite activities can be adapted to your needs and limitations, whether it's golf, swimming, walking, skiing, kayaking, gardening, or playing pickleball. If your old favorites become impossible, for whatever reason, the door is open for you to explore new activities that you might never have tried before, simply because you never had to. Now you may discover many fun and healthy options to increase your activity level.

"Now That I Can't Play Competitive Sports Anymore, the Fun Is Gone"

Once you've allowed yourself to grieve this loss, it's time to think about new ways to use your competitive spirit. Look for adaptive sports that allow you to compete on your own terms. Consider pickleball, which is played by young and old of all ability levels. Think about ways to compete with yourself as you work to improve your strength or endurance. Try out other competitive activities, such as board games or apps that allow you to play games while competing with others. Find ways to keep your competitive juices flowing.

"I Use a Wheelchair for Mobility, So Exercising Isn't an Option for Me"

Exercise comes in many varieties. The key components of a good exercise program include endurance training (aerobics), strength training (resistance), stretching (flexibility), and balance. All of these are possible whether you are seated or standing. A PT can teach you exercises that focus on your upper body while providing all of these benefits. For those whose mobility is very limited, exercises that promote leg strength, good seated posture, and healthy breathing can increase your comfort and reduce your fatigue. For those who are unable to exercise without assistance, the PT can teach a partner, friend, or paid helper how to help you stretch, work on your posture, and exercise your limbs.

"I Know Being Active Is Good for Me, but I Just Can't Get Motivated"

Motivation can be a barrier for any of us. Some days we feel energized, and some days we do not. Here are some tips to help you get started or stay on track:

- Ask yourself whether your mood might be getting in the way. Depression, which is very common in MS, can making everything feel impossible and uninteresting (see Chapter 7).
- Find an exercise buddy to make your activities more fun and interesting.
- Join an adaptive exercise class online or in person. (See Appendix 2 for exercise resources.)

"My Partner and I Can't Enjoy Physical Activities Together Anymore"

You and your partner can continue to enjoy many activities together—you may just need to do them a little differently. For example, you can use a **motorized scooter** to cover long distances in a museum, mall, or park and then walk together for as long as you're comfortable and safe. Then you can ride your scooter while your partner trots alongside you getting valuable exercise. Adaptive equipment for golf, skiing, kayaking, cycling, and other sports can allow you to enjoy these fun activities together.

Summary

The current recommendation—based on input from clinical and research experts in MS, rehabilitation, and physical activity—is at least 150 minutes of exercise and/or 150 minutes of lifestyle physical activity per week. Regardless of your ability level, you are already engaging in more activity than you realize—and you can do more. PTs and OTs can guide you in ways to stay active—or become more active—that are safe, enjoyable, and beneficial for you. Staying active is good not only for your physical health but also for your mood, cognitive functioning, and your MS.

CHAPTER 12

Diet and Nutrition

In this chapter, you will learn:

- The relationship between the immune system, nervous system, and gut microbiome
- The ways in which diet may affect multiple sclerosis
- The impact of diet on other health conditions that can impact the multiple sclerosis disease course
- Diets that have been studied in multiple sclerosis
- General dietary recommendations that may benefit a person with multiple sclerosis

One of the most exciting developments in neurology research is the recognition of the importance of diet in managing neurologic diseases. Although there is no diet that has been proven in large, well-controlled, clinical trials to change the course of multiple sclerosis (MS), there is growing evidence about the relationship between what we eat, the immune system, and the central nervous system (CNS).

The Interactivity of the Immune System, the Central Nervous System, and Gut Microbiota

We know from Chapter 1 that MS represents an attack by immune cells on the CNS. The immune system causes inflammation directed at cells and tissue within the CNS. This damages the CNS and produces many symptoms and a high risk for disability.

The immune system and the nervous system interact directly with each other. In addition, both interact with the bacteria in the gut (gastrointestinal tract), known as the gut microbiota (trillions of bacteria, viruses, and other microorganisms that live in the gut). The interaction between these systems is called the **gut–brain axis**. Signaling between these systems is done by chemical messengers or **neurotransmitters**. The gut microbiota influences the types and amount of chemical signaling that go to the various systems.

Of importance, the gut microbiota is not static; it is influenced by the foods we eat, as well as by smoking (bad), exercise (good), and our genetic makeup, infections, medications, and vitamin D levels. In other words, what we put into our bodies and how we treat our bodies influence how our bodies function and our overall health.

In MS, researchers hypothesize that changes in the gut microbiota may increase pro-inflammatory chemicals (**cytokines**) and stimulate a more inflammatory immune system. The hallmark of early MS is inflammation within the CNS, which means that a more inflammatory immune system may cause more MS damage. Research has shown that metabolism of the foods we eat plays a direct role in how immune cells function. **Saturated fats** (fats from animal sources such as beef, lamb, port, and full-fat daily products, which are solid at room temperature) and **trans fats** (mostly artificially produced fats that have no nutritional value) have been linked to increased inflammation, whereas **polyunsaturated fatty acid (PUFAs)**, which are liquid at room temperature, include healthy fats found in foods such as fish [salmon, herring, tuna, and trout], vegetable oils, walnuts, and flax seeds, PUFAs are thought to reduce inflammation.

The foods that we eat can also increase or decrease the risk of vascular comorbidities, including diabetes, high blood pressure, and high cholesterol. Obesity, which contributes to the risk of developing these vascular conditions, can also impact MS directly, in part due to the inflammatory cytokines that are produced by fatty tissue. A diet high in saturated fats, salt, refined sugars, and excessive calories increases risk for vascular comorbidities, whereas a diet lower in saturated fats, salt, refined sugars, and calories can reduce the risk of these conditions. Research has demonstrated that vascular comorbidities are more common in people with MS than the general population and that these conditions hasten disease progression and impact long-term outcomes. Therefore, a "healthy" diet that prevents or reduces the risk of these conditions indirectly affects the MS disease course. Let's look at the work that has been done to define healthy eating for a person with MS.

Diets Researched in Multiple Sclerosis

In general, the research on diets in MS has been focused on pro-inflammatory versus anti-inflammatory foods. Dietary components that appear to promote inflammation include saturated fats, trans fats, and highly refined starches and sugars. High-salt foods may also contribute to inflammation; however, their role in MS is not clear. They do, however, contribute to comorbidities such as high blood pressure. Let's look at a few of the diets that have been studied in MS, bearing in mind that there is no evidence that any diet by itself can change the MS disease course.

Wahls Protocol

The Wahls protocol was developed by Dr. Terry Wahls following her own diagnosis of MS. She found, through her own research, that strict adherence to a specific diet seemed to improve her mobility. Dr. Wahls believes supporting the mitochondria that produce energy in cells can be beneficial in MS. A modified version of the Paleo diet (eaten by our ancestors before grain farming and processed foods) forms the basis of this protocol. In the Wahls modified Paleo diet, eggs are excluded (allowed in the Paleo diet), and soy milk and gluten-free grains are permitted (not allowed in the Paleo diet).

Foods to eat include

- specific amounts of foods such as grass-fed meats;
- wild-caught fish;
- plenty of dark leafy green vegetables; and
- brightly colored fruits.

Foods to avoid are

- most grains;
- processed foods;
- soy;
- dairy;
- eggs; and
- beans.

One small, uncontrolled study found that a modified Paleo diet in combination with exercise and electrical muscle stimulation in people with secondary progressive MS demonstrated reduced fatigue. In a study comparing the Swank diet (see below) and the modified Paleo diet in people with relapsing–remitting MS, fatigue and physical quality of life were improved in both groups, whereas emotional quality of life scores improved only in the modified Paleo group. Because the Wahls diet excludes some food groups, it might result in nutritional deficiencies if appropriate supplements are not taken.

Swank Diet

Dr. Roy Swank developed this diet in 1990 to treat his MS patients. Foods to eat include

- whole-grain cereals and pasta;
- two cups each of fruits and vegetables per day;
- white fish and shellfish;

- skinned and trimmed poultry in any amount;
- dairy products with less than 1% fat; and
- cod liver oil and a multivitamin supplement.

Foods to avoid are

- red meat for 1 year, followed by no more than 3 oz. weekly;
- saturated fat intake less than 15 grams per day;
- unsaturated fat/oils intake below 20–50 grams per day; and
- processed foods containing saturated fats.

Swank's observational study over 20 years suggested that the diet reduced relapses, accumulation of disability, and mortality. However, his study was not controlled, and no standardized scoring system for disability was available at that time. Recently, the Wahls (a modified Paleo diet) and Swank diets were both found to reduce fatigue in people with MS.

Mediterranean Diet

The Mediterranean diet, which emphasizes consumption of whole grains, fresh fruits and vegetables, and lean proteins, has been studied extensively in the field of cardiac health and in MS.

Foods to eat include

- whole grains;
- vegetables;
- fruits;
- legumes;
- olive oil and other unsaturated oils, including sunflower, safflower, and rapeseed, among others;
- nuts and seeds;
- fish;

- poultry; and
- moderate but regular intake of alcohol (red wine with meals).

Foods to limit or avoid are

- saturated fats (primarily butter and animal fats);
- red meat; and
- dairy products.

Research on the Mediterranean diet in people with MS has shown less self-reported fatigue, better thinking (cognitive function), reduced depression and anxiety, and fewer MS symptoms overall.

Intermittent Fasting

Intermittent fasting is about when you eat rather than what you eat. Many regimens are available, but none should be undertaken without speaking with your health care provider first:

- A daily schedule restricts eating to a 6- to 8-hour period while fasting the remaining hours.
- A weekly schedule involves regular eating 5 days a week and eating one 500- to 600-calorie meal on each of the other 2 days.
- A restricted calorie regimen involves eating fewer calories than needed each day.

Individuals with diabetes, high blood pressure, eating disorders, and women who are pregnant or breastfeeding should not engage in any of the regimens. This type of diet, however, does not cause nutritional deficiencies as long as the foods that are eaten have nutritional value. For example, eating fast food when eating is allowed would not provide sufficient nutrients and would include foods that increase cardiovascular risks with excessive saturated fats, salt, and refined carbohydrates (white bread). There is limited evidence for the benefits of intermittent fasting or calorie restriction for people with MS. There is some evidence from animal studies that intermittent fasting may help reduce the immune effects of MS, and a few small studies in humans have reported improvement in some symptoms and immune parameters. More research is needed to determine the benefits and risks for people with MS.

Gluten-Free Diet

In addition to the previously discussed diets, the gluten-free (GF) diet has received attention by the MS community. Gluten is a major component of wheat proteins and is also found in rye and barley. People with celiac disease have certain antibodies to this protein and cannot tolerate any gluten. The GF diet contains no wheat, barley, rye, or triticales (a cross between wheat and rye). It is the recommended diet for people with celiac disease and for people who have an established sensitivity to gluten. The prevalence of true gluten sensitivity in the general population is about 6%, and the prevalence of celiac disease is about 0.5–1%.

There is currently no evidence to suggest that a GF diet is beneficial to the MS disease process or MS symptoms. In addition, there is no evidence that supports a connection between gluten and MS. However, there are many people, with and without MS, who feel better when following a GF diet. When following a GF or other diet, it is important to be sure the diet is meeting your nutritional needs with sufficient proteins, carbohydrates, fats, vitamins, and fiber. A GF diet may have deficiencies in iron, fiber, B vitamins, vitamin D, calcium, phosphorous, and zinc.

Vitamin D

Research has also been conducted on dietary supplements, and most extensively on vitamin D. Vitamin D is actually a hormone and important for the absorption of calcium, which is critical for bone health. Vitamin D is also present in immune cells and enhances anti-inflammatory activity. Low vitamin D has been established as a risk factor for the development of MS but not the cause of MS. However, despite multiple clinical trials, vitamin D supplementation is not established as helpful to the MS disease course or symptom management. A 2023 study of vitamin D supplementation found no impact on MS relapses, and other research studies have not shown benefit on disease progression, relapses, or magnetic resonance imaging outcomes.

Other Dietary Supplements

Various clinical research studies on supplements including biotin (vitamin B_7), vitamin A, coenzyme Q10, and others have not demonstrated any significant benefit for MS or MS symptoms. Early clinical trials on biotin suggested a role in progressive MS; however, in larger clinical trials, the results were not as favorable. Limited data suggest that omega-3 fatty acids, which are found in fatty fish and many nuts and seeds, may have some anti-inflammatory properties.

What Is a Healthy Diet for Multiple Sclerosis?

While many different dietary strategies are being promoted for people with MS, there is currently insufficient evidence to suggest that any of these change the MS disease course. However, these diets do have certain things in common, including reduced intake of processed foods, highly refined sugars, starches, and food that is high in saturated fat. And virtually all of these diets recommend increased consumption of whole grains and colorful fruits and vegetables. To date, there appears to be the most robust evidence for following a Mediterranean-type diet. This kind of healthy eating may prolong life, can reduce the risk of comorbid health conditions that can increase the risk of MS progression, and may improve some MS symptoms and function.

While you may want to follow optimal diet recommendations, you may encounter MS-related or other barriers to doing so. MS fatigue may challenge your efforts to prepare healthy meals from scratch, making it easier to just throw a processed meal in the microwave. Physical impairments such as loss of dexterity may also make it more difficult to cook. There may be financial barriers to obtaining healthy foods such as fresh fruits and vegetables. Or you may be confused as to what exactly a "healthy" diet looks like.

A nutritionist or registered dietician can provide information about what foods are best to eat and suggest healthy ways to prepare them. An occupational therapist can suggest strategies and tools that make shopping and meal preparation easier. One simple example is to do a lot of meal prep on a "good day" when you have lots of energy and freeze most of what you cook for future meals. When feasible, prepared meal delivery services can provide nutritious "heat and eat" meals or simple-to-prepare meal kits. If you have trouble obtaining fresh fruits and vegetables, frozen and some canned foods are just as nutritious while being more available and less expensive.

Additional resources on supplements can be found in Appendix 2.

CHAPTER 13

Relationships and Communication

In this chapter, you will learn:

- The qualities that characterize meaningful and lasting relationships
- The ways that a chronic, unpredictable illness can impact relationships with partners and spouses, children, parents, and close friends
- Recommended strategies for maintaining healthy and comfortable relationships
- Tips for ways to listen and talk with care and intent

Our important relationships evolve and grow over time, adapting to individual needs and shared circumstances. We anticipate many of the life changes that occur for all of us, but multiple sclerosis (MS) feels like an unwelcome and frightening intrusion into even the strongest relationships.

Healthy, Satisfying Relationships Have a Few Things in Common

Whether we're talking about couples, parents and children, or close friends, the healthiest relationships are based on

- mutual trust and respect;
- support for one another's goals and priorities;

- openness and honesty;
- caring and warmth;
- shared problem-solving; and
- help and assistance when needed.

Although MS is most commonly diagnosed in young adults, it can also occur in young children and older adults, which means that relationships across the life span can be impacted. You may be dealing with a child, a parent, or a spouse who has MS. Or you may be a person with MS who is trying to help your partner, children, parents, or close friends understand the changes that MS brought to your life. Regardless of the type of relationship, these core values apply. So, how can you manage your relationships optimally in the face of MS challenges?

Multiple Sclerosis Is a "We Disease" and Not a "Me Disease"

As discussed in Chapter 10 for support partners, when one person in a family is diagnosed with MS, the entire family lives with its presence. Although the person with MS is experiencing the symptoms and discomforts of MS, family members live with the impact as well, and they share feelings of anxiety, sadness, and anger. Partners may have feelings of guilt—one for having a disease that impacts family life and the other for being healthy while their loved one lives with MS. Other family members, particularly elderly parents and young children, may also feel guilty, wondering what they did to make this happen.

Accurate, age-appropriate information about MS will help calm fears, promote open communication, and allow the whole family to become part of the support team. Everyone has questions and worries, and the information can help them formulate their questions and feel more comfortable asking them. MS advocacy organizations (Can Do

MS, the National Multiple Sclerosis Society, the Multiple Sclerosis Association of America, and the Multiple Sclerosis Foundation) offer free information about MS for people of all ages.

Consider How Your Important Relationships May Be Affected

Regardless of the type of relationship(s) you and your support partner(s) have, it is helpful to think about the ways it has evolved since the MS diagnosis.

Spouse/Partner

Most couples settle into a rhythm over time: a set of shared goals, fairly predictable daily routine, and mutually agreeable assignment of chores and responsibilities. When one person is diagnosed with MS, the rhythm may be thrown off sporadically or more consistently. Responsibilities may need to be shifted, schedules may be disrupted, and shared plans and goals may be thrown off the rails. Partners need to share the feelings of sadness, anxiety, and anger that may be overwhelming at times. The better they are able to support one another through the emotional turmoil, the better they are able to begin adapting and problem-solving together.

Relationships work best when each person feels like a valued partner. When one person's MS makes their traditional role in the partnership difficult or impossible, a shift takes place, which may result in one partner doing less and the other doing more. This works fine on a temporary basis but doesn't wear well over time. If the person with MS has to give up some tasks or responsibilities, it's important for them to take on different ones that they are able to manage. These changes tend to evolve more smoothly when partners talk about them proactively and honestly. Keep in mind that changing responsibilities can cause conflict, which makes open dialogue about balanced task distribution all the more important. Ultimately, the goal is for each partner to contribute to the household in whatever ways they can. This not only allows the household to function but also ensures that both partners feel valued, respected, and cared for.

The best possible outcome is one that allows MS to get the attention and resources it needs without giving it more than necessary. It has often been said that "MS is greedy"—that it will take all the time and attention it can get. The goal is to keep it in its place—dealing with it, adapting to its presence, and getting on with life in ways that allow the partnership to remain on an even keel, ensuring that each person's needs are met.

Elderly Parents

"Once a parent, always a parent" is a truism. Parents don't stop worrying or wanting to help just because their children are now adults. Keeping them informed about how you're doing and how they can help is important, particularly if they live far away and can't see you in person very often. It's a good idea to come up with a plan together about how often you'll communicate and how all of you can stay current with your health issues and theirs. Every family does this a bit differently, but having a shared plan helps everyone worry less and support each other more effectively.

Some adults with MS may decide not to share information about their diagnosis with aging parents. While their intention is to protect their parents from worry, the unintended result may be to create barriers to communication and connection. Parents have a way of sensing when something is bothering their children or not going well in their lives. The best strategy may be to share information about the MS diagnosis, along with reassurance that you are getting the care you need and will keep them updated on things are going.

Parents (and other family members) sometimes try to help by providing you with a lot of advice, some of it good and some of it quite misguided. The best way to handle this situation is to assure them that you are working with a health care team that is taking good care of you and that you are keeping up with the latest MS news through MS advocacy organizations.

Adult Children of a Person with Multiple Sclerosis

Members of the "sandwich generation"—those who take care of aging parents as well as children of their own—often feel overwhelmed, exhausted, and guilt-ridden about not being able to give the people they love as much care and attention as they would like to. Adults who find themselves in this situation can get helpful suggestions and support from the MS advocacy organizations as well as from support groups or other resources in their community. What's most important is to recognize that you don't have to do it alone.

Parent of a Child with Multiple Sclerosis

Although most people are diagnosed with MS between ages 20 and 40 years, children younger than age 16 years make up approximately 3–5% of people with MS, with many more diagnosed in their late teens. The pediatric MS resources provided in Appendix 2 offer information about the diagnosis and management of pediatric MS, strategies for working with your child's school, ways to partner with your child's health care team, and tips for negotiating adolescence (always a challenging time) in a child who is balancing the need for your care and support with their need for autonomy. Parents of children with MS have formed large support networks to problem-solve and support one another. In addition, the National Multiple Sclerosis Society offers information, support, and recreational activities for children, as well as camps for families living with MS. Seeking support for your child is as beneficial as the support you get for yourself.

Extended Family and Friends

While some people with MS find that their extended family and friends provide support, assistance, and a reassuring presence, others find their circle dwindling as friends or family fade away. If you're fortunate to have support from those around you, let them know you appreciate it and be specific in the ways that they can help you the most (e.g., "Could you drive me to the doctor on Thursday at 2:00?" "When you go to the store, could you pick up these items for me?" and "Could you watch the kids for 2 hours on Saturday while I take a nap?"). Most people want to be helpful but have no way to know what you need unless you tell them.

Many of those who shy away simply don't know what to say or do when they hear about your diagnosis or a recent relapse. Some even worry that it may be contagious. The more time that passes without saying or doing anything, the more awkward it feels for them to reach out. It's worth your while to risk reaching out to them—saying that you miss them, would like to find a way to connect, and that you'd be happy to explain MS or answer any questions they may have.

Communication Is the Key

We communicate all the time in a variety of ways: words, emails, texts, social media, body language, and behavior. In fact, we're communicating even when we don't realize it. For relationships to thrive, communication needs to be thoughtful and intentional so that we effectively convey what we mean, allow the other person to do the same, and truly listen to one another. Unfortunately, many obstacles can get in the way:

- No good time or place for an extended conversation
- Concerns about upsetting or worrying the other person

- Inability to express angry thoughts or feelings in a constructive way
- Topics that feel too sensitive or difficult to put into words
- Differences in the way individuals express themselves (the "talker" vs. the "doer")

Make communication a priority. Schedule time for important conversations and make sure that you are in a distraction-free environment so that you both can focus. Particularly if you're experiencing memory or attention problems due to MS (or aging), eliminating distractions will help you hear and remember important conversations. We encourage you and your support partner(s) to pay attention to your body language. Eye-rolling, looking at your phone, flipping through TV channels, shoulder-shrugging, rolling over and going to sleep, and other dismissive behaviors leave the other person feeling hurt and unheard. The best conversations start with listening:

- Make eye contact.
- Turn toward the person you're talking with.
- Confirm what you've heard.
- Be patient; it may take the other person time to convey their thoughts and feelings.
- Try not to interrupt or finish the other person's sentence, even if you feel impatient.
- If you need time to think about what's been said and how to respond, say so—but let the other person know when you'll respond.

Talk with thought and care; the words you use matter:

- Think before you speak to avoid hurt or misunderstanding.
- Give the other person time to think and respond.

- Avoid starting sentences with "You always . . ." or "You never . . ."—phrases that tend put the other person on the defensive.
- Approach sensitive topics with sensitivity.

Topics such as sexual function, bowel and bladder problems, cognitive changes, and the unpredictable future, to name a few, can make people uncomfortable enough that they shy away from talking about them at all. But managing these issues that impact both of you requires sharing feelings and solutions. The MS advocacy groups offer brochures, webinars, and educational programs to help you address these issues. In addition to providing the information, these resources give you the vocabulary you may need to jumpstart the conversations more comfortably. Your MS provider can also be a very helpful resource, or they can refer you to someone else who can support you, such as a nurse or mental health professional.

Do not try to problem-solve when you're in the middle of an argument. No one thinks clearly, reaches compromise, or finds solutions when they're in a rage. Agree to talk again when tempers have cooled. Share your perspectives and look for common ground or possible compromise. And work with a counselor or therapist if you're finding it difficult to jumpstart tough conversations or resolve conflict.

The best relationships take time and effort. Many couples living with MS say that managing the disease together has brought them closer—forced them to improve their communication and truly listen to one another. For those who find it more difficult, help is available.

Summary

Everyone in the family lives with MS—it is definitely a "we disease" rather than a "me disease." Whether it's a spouse or partner, parent, child, or close friend, effective relationships are based on mutual trust and respect, support for one another's goals and priorities, and effective and thoughtful communication. Effective problem-solving and mutual support start with open and honest conversations, fueled by caring and warmth.

CHAPTER 14

Intimacy and Sexuality

In this chapter, you will learn:

- Ways that multiple sclerosis can impact sexuality and intimacy
- Tips for talking about the changes that may occur
- How couples can manage these challenges
- Treatment strategies that are available to help
- How to get the help you need

Intimacy means different things to different people. For some, it's more about closeness, connection, trust, and warmth, which they experience in a variety of relationships in their lives. For others, being intimate is about being sexual, with physical intimacy being the primary way they feel closeness with another person. Some people need to feel intimate before they can connect sexually with another person, while others need to connect sexually to feel the safety and warmth of intimacy. This chapter is for all of you.

Multiple sclerosis (MS) can impact relationships, shift roles, and affect people's efforts to communicate effectively with one another (see Chapter 13). These kinds of changes can affect not only daily interactions and activities but also the intimate connections that people develop over time. Feelings, worries, and reactions to the unpredictable changes of MS may make it more difficult for people to connect and communicate. When this happens, it can affect an intimate sexual relationship as well, creating a feeling of distance or uncertainty. Along with its potential impact on emotional intimacy, MS can also have a significant impact on sexual feelings and responses, which in turn can also affect a couple's feelings of closeness and connection. In other words, emotional and physical intimacy interact in complex ways.

How Multiple Sclerosis Can Impact Sexual Feelings and Responses

Most people with MS will experience some changes in sexual function. These changes have been categorized as primary, secondary, and tertiary sexual dysfunction.

Primary Sexual Dysfunction

Primary sexual problems are caused by inflammation and damage to nerve pathways in the brain and spinal cord that disrupt transmission of messages within the central nervous system and affect feelings, sensation, and physical function throughout the body. When this occurs, a person may notice several different changes, including a loss of sexual desire (**libido**). Women more often than men report a lessening or loss of the spark they once had. It has been described by many as "a light switch got turned off" or "I'm just not into it anymore." This sudden lack of interest can be puzzling and confusing to both partners and feels like a major loss. As discussed in Chapter 7, grieving is a normal and healthy reaction to any loss, and this is no different. The feelings need to be acknowledged and processed over time. Men often experience reduced arousal and have difficulty achieving or maintaining an erection, whereas women tend to experience reduced vaginal lubrication.

Other primary sexual symptoms include changes in orgasm intensity or difficulty reaching orgasm, which are common in both women and men, as well as sensory changes such as numbness, tingling, or pain. These sensory changes can interfere with sexual feelings and responses for both men and women, particularly when they occur in the genital area. Things that used to feel pleasurable may now feel painful, irritating, or like nothing at all.

Secondary Sexual Dysfunction

Secondary sexual problems are caused by other symptoms of MS as well as some of the medications a person may be taking. For example, MS fatigue can move sexual activity way down a person's priority list. Nerve pain (neuropathic pain) can cause even the slightest touch to be uncomfortable or even excruciating, and stiffness related to spasticity can make sexual positions difficult or impossible. Many people report that sexual activity or orgasm can cause painful spasms in their legs or torso. Bladder or bowel issues can make people anxious about having an accident during sex, and depression can make a person feel disinterested in sex. Medications, including some antidepressants, bladder medications, blood pressure medications, and statins, among others, can affect sexual function, as can hormonal changes related to menopause and normal aging.

Tertiary Sexual Dysfunction

Tertiary sexual problems are less specific than the primary or secondary problems yet may pose even greater challenges for intimate relationships. The media make it clear that all of us should be healthy, young, active, and ready and willing for sex at any time—all of which flies in the face of the realities of MS and real life. But this messaging still impacts us. The farther a person feels from that unrealistic standard, the more unattractive or unaroused they may feel. Changes in self-image and self-esteem related to MS can make people feel less desirable, attractive, and confident. Negative attitudes about illness and disability may interfere with a support partner's interest, cause them anxiety about hurting or tiring their partner, or make them feel guilty about wanting sexual activity when their partner is less interested. With all these factors in play, it can be challenging to know how to get this important part of your life to a more comfortable and pleasurable place. Let's take it a step at a time.

Step 1: Communicating with Each Other About What's Going On

For most people, sex is very difficult to talk about. We tend not to have comfortable words for it, our expectations and wishes can blind us to another person's feelings or needs, and we tend to jump to conclusions about things when we really need to be listening and talking. Reading this chapter and other materials (see Appendix 2) helps both of you understand the changes that can occur with MS and will give you the words you need to start the conversation. And don't be afraid to be open and honest about what has changed—and how you each feel about it—to avoid misconceptions (e.g., "He doesn't find me attractive anymore," "She's having an affair," "He's turned off by my MS," or "She thinks I'm less of a man now") and to allow you to begin some shared problem-solving strategies.

Step 2: Talking to Your Health Care Provider

If you haven't already been asked about sexual function during your regular visits, bring it up. If your provider seems uncomfortable talking about it, perhaps it is time to search for a different provider. Nurses, mental health professionals, and rehabilitation professionals (physical therapists and occupational therapists) can all be immensely helpful.

Changes in sexual function are a common symptom of MS that deserves the same care and attention as your other symptoms, which means that you need to advocate for yourself. If you need to schedule an extra appointment just to talk about this issue, then do it. Be specific with your questions. You and your provider will need to look for the best strategies to address your primary, secondary, and tertiary challenges and identify the members of the health care team—whether it be a nurse, a rehabilitation professional, a mental health professional, or a sex therapist—who can help you.

Step 3: Understanding and Exploring Your Management Options

Let your health care team know what you need. You and your partner are the captains of this treatment team, which means that you will be letting the other members of the team know what you want and need in the way of help. Start by examining your attitudes and feelings with one another. If your intimate connection, including your sexual life, is important to you both, you have the chance to begin looking at how to adapt to whatever changes MS is causing. Like every other aspect of your life that's impacted by MS, you'll find that you can do some of your preferred activities a little differently (e.g., with a little more planning, changes in timing or positioning, a modification of some medications, and preemptive trips to the bathroom to avoid accidents).

If these adaptations don't do the trick, it's time to look for different ways to give and receive pleasure that you both enjoy. Try a **body mapping exercise**, which gives you a private opportunity to get to know your body really well (what feels good and what doesn't, which parts like to be touched, what kinds of touch feel best, and what nonsexual body parts like to be stroked or rubbed), and then teach your partner. Personal exploration by yourself comes first, followed by time together to teach and learn. This is a perfect way to share very personal information, which in itself is an important act of intimacy. Care partners can do the same—teaching their partner with MS how to give the greatest pleasure within the limits of their energy and physical abilities.

Do not be afraid to experiment with different treatment options. Physical therapists can help with positioning, use of pillows, and other strategies to promote your comfort. Both men and women can benefit from pelvic floor physical therapy. This subspecialty of physical therapy works to strengthen the pelvic floor muscle, which can help with both sexual functioning and bladder problems.

Medications may be helpful for arousal problems as well as managing other MS symptoms that get in your way. Men have access to an array of oral medications for erectile dysfunction. Most work well for about 50% of men with MS. Urologists—who treat bladder problems (see Chapter 8) as well as male sexual dysfunction—can offer other options if the oral medications don't work well for you. There are also medications and devices for women that can help with low arousal. Your gynecologist is probably your best source of information about these treatment strategies. To help with vaginal lubrication, use an over-the-counter, water-based lubricant—and use it generously.

For people who have lost sensitivity in their genital area, more stimulation may be needed. Oral sex, manual sex, vibrators, and other toys can all offer greater stimulation than intercourse. Being open and creative will help you find your own solutions.

Nerve pain is generally managed with medication (see Chapter 6). However, the medications most commonly used to treat nerve pain can cause significant fatigue, so talk with your provider about dosing and timing. Medications that manage spasticity can be timed to allow for maximum flexibility and comfort during sexual activity. Bladder medications (see Chapter 8) can be very drying, contributing to the discomfort of vaginal dryness. Discuss medication options with your provider to ensure you're taking a medication that allows maximum comfort. If you do intermittent self-catheterization, catheterizing just before sexual activity can eliminate the worry about bladder accidents.

Step 4: Revisiting Your Attitudes and Preconceived Ideas

Sexual feelings and responses change for a variety of reasons over the course of a lifetime. Normal aging, menopause, and other acute or chronic illnesses and their treatments can all affect the way we and our bodies respond. Allow yourself the luxury of revamping some of your ideas.

We have all been taught that orgasm is the be-all and end-all of sex, but if orgasm becomes difficult or impossible, there are other ways to feel intense pleasure. By focusing more on the process rather than just the end goal, you can discover a myriad of pleasures that you hadn't even thought about before. We're not saying that losing one's ability to experience an orgasm isn't a loss—it is a loss that one grieves over and misses. But it isn't the end of sexuality or sexual pleasure.

Maintaining intimacy and pleasure in your relationship over a lifetime takes flexibility, creativity, and a sense of humor. Trying to do old things in new ways can be fun, exciting, and pleasurable—you just need to open yourselves up to the possibilities when the old ways aren't working for you. And you don't need to be in synch all the time. One of you can feel and be sexual while the other watches or caresses or hugs. You may not always be in sync, and that's OK, as long as each person's feelings and needs are respected.

Romance is all in the mind—and your mind can do amazing things. Think about what helps you relax and feel cozy and close, and what turns your mind on. Letting yourself take the time to enjoy the moment, engage in comfortable caresses, and feel close can give your body time to catch up. Sometimes you need to start on faith, even when you don't feel like it, because your body is slower than it used to be to respond. Give it a little time and patience. Use external cues to help build the romance. Music, lighting, a sexy movie that appeals to both of you, a sex toy or two—anything that both of you find pleasurable and appealing is worth trying.

As you work through these changes and challenges together, you'll find your intimacy growing in ways you had never anticipated.

Summary

Intimacy and sexuality are an important part of our lives. Regardless of our age, race, gender, sexual orientation, or relationship status, we deserve to get help with challenges we encounter. MS can affect sexual function and feelings in a variety of ways. Some (primary) changes are caused directly by inflammatory damage in the spinal cord and brain. Other (secondary) changes are caused by MS symptoms such as fatigue, pain, spasticity, bladder or bowel problems, or the medications taken to manage MS symptoms and other health conditions. Still other (tertiary) changes are caused by attitudes and feelings about disability and sexuality. Your health care team can help you address all of these, but the help begins with you raising your questions and concerns. For more resources on sexuality and intimacy, see Appendix 2.

CHAPTER 15

Reproductive and Parenting Issues

In this chapter, you will learn:

- How pregnancy affects the multiple sclerosis disease course and how having multiple sclerosis affects pregnancy
- How multiple sclerosis treatments affect contraception and fertility
- How conception, pregnancy, and the postpartum period impact the timing of multiple-sclerosis disease-modifying therapies
- How multiple sclerosis is likely to impact parenting
- What is known about the impact of menopause on multiple sclerosis

The majority of people who develop multiple sclerosis (MS) are young adults in their 20s and 30s; more than two-thirds of them are women. Thoughts about starting or enlarging their families are top of mind for many—and even those who are not planning to have children are generally sexually active. In this chapter, we address the most common questions about pregnancy, contraception, and fertility.

It was previously thought that women with MS should not have children because pregnancy would worsen the disease or increase disability or that parenting would be too taxing or challenging for parents with MS. This is definitely not the case. We have since learned that women with MS do very well during pregnancy and delivery and that a person with MS can raise healthy and happy children.

Multiple Sclerosis and Pregnancy

Many studies have documented that women with MS can conceive, give birth, and nurse their babies just as other women do. Women with MS face the same reproductive risks and challenges that all women face, but there are additional concerns that are specific to MS.

People with MS do not have more fertility challenges than those without MS and must pay the same attention to contraceptive choices as anyone else. Pregnancy, labor, and delivery in women with MS are the same as they are in women with comparable general and obstetric health, and rates of children with birth defects are the same for women with MS and the general population. However, there is some evidence that women with MS may give birth to babies with a slightly lower than average birth weight. Women generally feel well during pregnancy, although some MS symptoms—including urinary frequency or urgency, fatigue, or difficulty walking—are likely to increase problems that are already common in pregnant women.

Women with spinal cord lesions that produce weakness in the legs may have more difficulty pushing during delivery and may require additional assistance. Epidural and general anesthesia are considered safe, as are cesarean sections when they are needed.

Most of the medications used to treat MS symptoms, such as bladder problems or muscle spasticity, are avoided during pregnancy because they are known to be, or could possibly be, unsafe for the developing fetus. Therefore, MS symptoms are generally managed with strategies other than drugs, including rehabilitation techniques and strategies such as intermittent catheterization.

Pregnancy Mimics the Actions of Disease-Modifying Therapies

As discussed in Chapter 1, MS represents an overactive and misdirected immune system that is attacking the central nervous system. The disease-modifying therapies (DMTs) that are prescribed to help manage the MS disease course reduce this immune response (see Chapter 3). Similarly, the changes that occur in a woman's body during pregnancy naturally alter or modulate the body's immune response. Let's look at how this occurs: A baby has one set of genes and proteins from its mother and one set from its father, which means that the mother's immune system would recognize the father's proteins in the developing fetus as "foreign" and attack them. Fortunately, the mother's immune system is modulated during pregnancy, so it does not recognize the fetus as foreign—which allows the fetus to grow and develop inside the mother's body. Research has shown that the natural immune modulation that occurs in all pregnant women reduces the relapse rate for women with MS by two-thirds compared with what it was prior to the pregnancy. As a result, many women with MS report feeling better while they are pregnant.

In women who had active disease with many relapses before becoming pregnant, there is a brief period of several months immediately after the baby is born when their relapse rate may be higher than before pregnancy. However, studies have also shown that while some women with MS who become pregnant may be more likely to have a relapse right after delivery, they do not have increased long-term disability compared with women with MS who do not become pregnant.

The end result is that DMTs are not as necessary during pregnancy, which is fortunate because almost all DMTs have been shown to cause harm to the fetus in animals or humans.

Managing Disease-Modifying Therapies Before and During Pregnancy

Multiple sclerosis care providers generally recommend stopping DMTs (see Chapter 3) for some period of time before attempting conception. The length of time depends on how long it takes the particular drug a woman is taking to completely leave her body, which generally ranges from a few weeks to several months. In the case of teriflunomide, it takes 2 years for the medication to leave the body completely. Both men and women need to stop this medication before trying to conceive. Your MS care provider may prescribe a medication to help lower the blood level of the medication more quickly.

A few DMTs in addition to teriflunomide may be present in semen as well, so men with MS should consult their MS care provider before trying to conceive. Some neurologists may allow a woman to continue taking beta-interferon or glatiramer acetate up until conception as these agents are thought to be safe. If you do become pregnant while on a DMT, let your MS provider know immediately.

The B cell depleting medications are generally cleared from the body within 3 or 4 months after administration and are not thought to cross the placenta until the second trimester. Remember that timing for conception and pregnancy should be raised with your MS care provider.

"**Rebound relapses**" during pregnancy have been reported in some women who were taking natalizumab (Tysabri) and fingolimod (Gilenya) prior to becoming pregnant. It is not clear whether the relapses occurred in these women because they stopped their medication or because they had a lot of disease activity before taking these medications. Rebound relapses have also been reported outside of pregnancy in adults who stopped these medications.

Managing Disease-Modifying Therapies Following Delivery

None of the DMTs are approved for use during breastfeeding (although there is some thought that nursing mothers may use B cell depleting medications—Rituxan, Ocrevus, and Kesimpta). Most providers will encourage a woman to breastfeed her baby if she wishes to do so. Breastfeeding itself does not appear to increase the risk of a relapse, and a few small studies suggest that exclusive breastfeeding for at least 2 months may even be somewhat protective against a post-partum relapse. Further research is needed in this area. However, if a woman had very active MS prior to becoming pregnant, her provider may suggest that she forgo breastfeeding so that she can resume treatment as quickly as possible and avoid an MS relapse. In this situation, the new mother can work with her MS care provider, partner, and pediatrician to determine the optimal time for her to resume her medication.

Jennifer and her husband went to see her neurologist a year ago because they were eager to start a family. The neurologist told Jennifer to stop her medication before trying to conceive. One month ago, Jennifer delivered a beautiful healthy daughter. Now she is experiencing some gait difficulty and imbalance. The neurologist examines Jennifer and finds some new weakness in her legs. The neurologist decides to treat this relapse with a short course of intravenous corticosteroids and some physical therapy, both of which are expected to improve Jennifer's ability to walk. Jennifer has been breastfeeding and will "pump and dump" while she is on steroids so as not to expose the baby to them.

Both the neurologist and Jennifer are concerned about her having another relapse, and so they agree that this may be a good time for Jennifer to stop breastfeeding and resume her previous DMT or consider switching to a higher efficacy medication.

The Risk of Multiple Sclerosis for a Child Whose Parent Has Multiple Sclerosis

Currently, there are no prenatal tests that can indicate whether a child whose parent or sibling has MS will develop the disease. While MS is not an inherited disease like Huntington's disease or cystic fibrosis, genes do play a role in the development of MS. Scientists have identified more than 200 genes that contribute to the overall risk of MS. The result is that the risk of developing MS in a first-degree relative (child or sibling) of someone with MS is about 4% compared with 0.5% in the general population.

Other Reproductive Issues

A person with MS may use any form of contraception. However, some of the medicines used for symptom management—particularly some of the anticonvulsant drugs used to treat pain and stimulants such as modafinil (Provigil) used to treat fatigue—may interfere with oral contraception, so it is a good idea to discuss alternative contraceptive options with your MS care provider. Women who have decreased dexterity in their hands may have difficulty using a barrier method such as a diaphragm.

Some women with MS may experience an increase in some of their neurologic symptoms right before their menstrual period, which resolve as soon as the period starts. It is not known what produces this increase in symptoms. Sometimes hormones are used to regulate periods to prevent this increased symptom activity. One report of a small number of patients suggests that aspirin may be useful in treating neurologic symptoms that occur around the time of a woman's period.

The effects of menopause on MS have not been extensively studied. Women with MS in general do not appear to reach menopause earlier or later than the general population. Many symptoms of MS, such as fatigue, bladder symptoms, cognitive issues, and mood changes, may be worsened by menopause. Currently, there are no data to indicate that taking hormone replacements to relieve menopausal symptoms is problematic for women with MS.

Parenting with Multiple Sclerosis

Parenting with or without MS is a joyful and challenging adventure for which most of us feel ill-equipped. Keep in mind that babies quickly grow into toddlers and then teens. Most prospective parents with MS focus on the challenges of bringing a newborn home from the hospital, but we encourage you to think beyond those early days. Consider how much help you have available, a new mother's need for rest, and the layout of your home for energy conservation and ease. But think also about the needs of an active toddler, the busy life of a school-age child, and the schedules and activities of teens. It takes planning to meet your own needs as a person living with MS as well as the needs of your child(ren). If you would like some guidance in this area, schedule an appointment with an occupational therapist or mental health professional to talk about any challenges you anticipate.

Children as young as toddlers feel the impact of a parent's MS. Even if the symptoms are invisible, children tune into tension, mood changes, and disruptions in everyday rhythms. They may ask why you're so tired, why you look sad, what's hurting you, why you're walking funny, or why you're so cranky. Children may also assume blame, wondering if their "bad" behavior has somehow caused this to happen.

While parents may think it best to protect their children from the MS by keeping it secret or making excuses for changes in plans, the best way to help children cope and adapt is to give them accurate information that's geared to their developmental level. Much like teaching children about sex or any other complex topic, it's wise to start by answering questions with very simple facts and then providing more detailed information as their questions become more sophisticated.

The most common questions on children's minds, regardless of their ages, are "Are you going to die?" "Will I catch it?" and "Did I cause it?" For the youngest children, the answers are "No," "No," and "No." As children grow into teens and young adults, you can provide more details about MS and the complex factors that determine a person's risk of getting MS and also the varying levels of disability that people may experience. And you can reassure children of any age that there is nothing they did that caused you to get MS. See Appendix 2 for resources on talking about MS with children and teens.

You and your children live with the unpredictability of MS symptoms. Some days you have more energy than others, your ability to function may change from day to day, and symptoms such as pain or urinary problems can interfere with the best-laid plans. Having a plan B for every plan A is your best strategy for avoiding disappointments. Take advantage of mobility devices to help you stay busy and active with your kids. This will not only ensure that you can participate with them in their activities but also demonstrate your creativity, flexibility, and ability to work around challenges you have.

And let your kids know how they can help. Children of parents with MS can grow up to be caring, responsible, confident adults who feel good about the ways they have contributed to the family. Trying to shield them from your MS deprives them of valuable opportunities to learn and grow into the kind of adult you want them to be.

Summary

Women and men with MS can have healthy, happy children. Your MS care provider can work with you to manage your MS before, during, and after pregnancy. Collaborate with your MS care provider, obstetrician, and pediatrician to ensure the best possible care for yourself and your newborn during pregnancy and after delivery. In addition to the challenges of parenting that everyone faces, parents with MS may have additional needs to be addressed with their MS care providers.

CHAPTER 16

Planning for the Future While Finding Meaning in the Present

In this chapter, you will learn:

- How to come to terms with this variability and unpredictability
- Strategies for taking charge of aspects of your life and your multiple sclerosis that are within your control
- How to find meaning and purpose after change and loss
- Steps you can take toward self-acceptance, adaptation, and continued growth

One of the first things people confront with multiple sclerosis (MS) is its unpredictability. Despite all the progress that has been made in diagnosing and treating this disease, no one can tell a person with MS exactly what the future is likely to hold for them. Each person's MS is different, with a range of possible symptoms that fluctuate from one day to the next and a disease course that behaves according to its own rules. The MS disease-modifying therapies (DMTs) impact the natural history of MS, but the course still varies from person to person. While MS is generally considered a progressive disease, the degree and speed of progression are highly variable. Some people will stay stable for years at a time, whereas others will experience disruptive and potentially disabling relapses or gradually progressive disability as time passes. This chapter presents some strategies to help you navigate the variability and uncertainty of life with MS.

Getting Your Head Around Unpredictability

For young adults who are just beginning their careers and families, the diagnosis of a chronic, unpredictable illness such as MS may be their first experience with health issues or physical changes that could challenge their plans and dreams. For many, this is the hardest part of the first few months or years of life with MS. The best way to deal with these feelings is to take action regarding the things that are within your control.

The DMTs discussed in Chapter 3 are your best tool for controlling the disease as much as possible and for protecting your future. Start treatment early and work with your MS care provider over time to ensure you are taking the best medication for your MS. This is your "ace in the hole." While it's not a guarantee, it's the best reassurance to be had at this time.

Managing your overall health and wellness is an important part of taking care of your MS. The following all contribute to living well with MS: getting adequate exercise and physical activity; enjoying a healthy diet; paying attention to your emotional, social, and spiritual well-being; and staying up-to-date with **preventive health screenings** and vaccinations. Taking these steps will position you to feel stronger and better able to manage the challenges of MS. It will also reduce comorbid health conditions, such as high blood pressure, high cholesterol, and diabetes, that can have a negative impact on your MS (see Chapter 9). Combining attention to your overall health and wellness with early and ongoing use of DMTs will form the strongest foundation for your care.

To feel and function at your best, advocate for yourself with your health care team to ensure that your symptoms are well managed and your emotional and cognitive functioning are evaluated on a regular basis. Time is limited with the health care team, so bring a prioritized list of your questions and concerns to your visits to help ensure that your priorities are addressed. Provide your MS care and primary care providers with your advance directives and health care proxy information (discussed below). In the event that you ever need to be hospitalized, the hospital is likely to ask for these documents upon admission. While these documents are unlikely to be needed in the near future, taking the time to think about your personal priorities and preferences will help you feel more secure.

These are all ways that you can feel more in control of your health and wellness now and in the future, which in turn will help you feel less vulnerable in the face of MS.

Building a Safety Net for Your Future

Your best bet is to approach the unpredictability of MS with a "prepare for the worst while hoping for the best" mindset. Planning for the best doesn't prepare for any possible bumps in the road, whereas planning for the worst sets you up to manage the bumps if and when they occur. So, take an honest look at your current worry list—the "what if this happens or that happens?" worries that feel overwhelming— and begin to think about some steps you could take today that would allow you to worry less and get on with living your life. Here are some examples:

- Talk with your MS care provider about your plans for starting or growing your family. Together, you and your provider can figure out the timing of your medications (see Chapter 15) and strategies for ensuring that you have the best pregnancy and childbirth experience.
- Take a look at the symptoms you're experiencing and the type of work you do. Many people with MS leave the workforce prematurely, with fatigue and cognitive issues being the most common reasons. Thinking proactively about your work situation can lay the groundwork for long-term, successful employment. Some types of careers are highly dependent on

physical abilities: mobility, agility, balance, and coordination. Others are more dependent on strong cognitive skills, clear thinking, and agile decision-making. It's never too early to consult with a speech–language pathologist about cognitive issues, a physical therapist about physical abilities, or an occupational therapist about general work concerns that may develop. An employment specialist can help you anticipate challenges you may experience on the job and identify the types of reasonable accommodations you might request from your employer. These conversations can help you increase your productivity on the job and enable you to stay in the workplace as long as you want and are able to. These conversations can also help you think about training for future career options in case you become unable to perform in your current profession. Knowing you have given thought to this will help you feel more prepared.

- Think about the community you live in. This may not be a concern when you are diagnosed, but if you choose to move or if your condition changes, you will want to ask yourself the following questions: Do you have access to the care you need? Is accessible transportation available? Can you easily get to the local stores you need? Are you more isolated than you would like to be? Do you have a support system where you live?
- Consider the home you live in. While this may not be a concern at the time of your diagnosis, changes may occur over time that can impact where you live. Ask yourself the following questions: Can you easily navigate your living space? Does the layout of your home allow you to conserve your energy and feel comfortable? Are you able to fully use your space, or are you restricted from using certain rooms because of decreased mobility? This kind of honest assessment can help you make proactive decisions about your housing.
- Take a good look at your finances. MS is an expensive disease. It's never too early to get your financial plan in place.

A financial advisor with expertise in disability and chronic illness can help you plan for your future. While thinking about finances and insurance issues is uncomfortable for most of us, the conversations you have now can help you initiate financial strategies today that will put your mind at ease and set you up for a more stable financial future. The National Multiple Sclerosis Society (1-800-344-4867) offers a free consultation with a financial advisor. When selecting your own financial advisor for this type of planning, look for someone who has specialized training and certification in planning for individuals with special needs. They will be able to guide you concerning government benefits, special needs trusts, and tax implications.

- Work with your attorney to write your advance directives. Advance directives are the legal documents you provide to your health care team that specify your health care choices if a time comes when you are too ill to decide. One form of an advance directive is a living will, in which you specify the medical treatments, procedures, and medications you do or do not want to receive if you're incapacitated and unable to speak for yourself. Keep in mind that different states have different definitions for these terms, so consulting with your state legislature and a local attorney can help ensure that you have the documents you need. A health care proxy is a document that names someone you trust as your proxy or agent to express your wishes and make health care decisions on your behalf. Your proxy or agent is guided by the wishes expressed in your living will. It's important to review these documents yearly to ensure they accurately reflect your wishes, your state of health, state of residence, marital status, and other major life factors. Identify the individual(s) who will have your financial power of attorney and medical power of attorney (your health care proxy). These individuals should be people you trust to carry out your wishes.

All of these strategies require you to look the unpredictable in the eye. We encourage you to take all the "What-ifs" that you worry about and turn them into strategies for feeling safer, less vulnerable, and more secure regardless of what MS brings your way. We know that getting a diagnosis of MS can shake your foundations, causing you to wonder why this happened, what it means for your life, and who you are now that the disease is bringing so many changes to your life. Keep reading—we have some ideas to help you with these feelings.

Life Is a Continuing Series of Snapshots in Time

Over our lifetimes, we all carry a picture of ourselves. The picture changes as we grow, evolve, and age, but our core identify remains remarkably consistent—the things we like about ourselves and those we work to develop or change, the personality traits that shape our relationships and roles, and the talents that inform our work and hobbies.

The diagnosis of MS or disease progression may call into question many things you have taken for granted about yourself and your life. You may see yourself differently and expect that others will see you differently. The plans and dreams you had for your life may seem less realistic or even impossible. And you may wonder how you will continue to make your mark, do your share, create or maintain important relationships, or stay engaged with the world around you. The goal is to find a way to incorporate the diagnosis of MS—and the physical, cognitive, or emotional changes it may bring—into your self-portrait, without losing sight of all the other parts of you that make you unique. Space will always be needed in your life for the demands MS makes on your time, energy, and attention, but the goal is to give it no more than it needs. We all need a strong foundation to move forward with our lives and meet challenges when they arise. If your life has been shaken to the core by MS changes, the first step is to rebuild that foundation.

Allow Yourself to Grieve Over the Changes and Losses

Healthy grieving (see Chapter 7 for more detail) is the first step toward letting go of what you had and moving toward a new future—from the way you saw yourself before your diagnosis to what you've learned about yourself since your MS diagnosis, and from what your goals were to how you might adapt them to the unpredictable changes of MS. This ability to see and do things differently is a challenging learning process that takes time.

Ask Yourself What Defines You

- What are your strengths and talents? Perhaps you are very wise or intuitive or flexible? Maybe you have a gift for painting, music, or building things?
- What are your core values? Are you all about fairness or inclusivity, honesty, or generosity? Self-sufficiency or teamwork?
- What are you passionate about? Maybe it's your family, your faith, the natural world, or the work you do?
- Where do your priorities lie? Are you particularly focused on your career path, raising your kids, or taking care of others?
- What would you like to accomplish? Do you have some long-term goals that have special meaning for you?
- What would you like to share with others? Perhaps you have talents, wisdom, gifts, or resources that you would like others to enjoy?

Each person's answers to these questions are different—yours are unique to you. You may want to ask yourself these same questions periodically to help you stay grounded in the face of MS challenges. If you get stuck and have difficulty coming up with answers, ask your partner or another important person in your life to help you.

Sometimes, they can see your talents, strengths, and values even when you're feeling out of touch with them or less confident about them. And if you find that MS symptoms are getting in the way of using the talents, skills, and passions that make you unique, consider working with an occupational therapist or a mental health professional to develop new or adapted ways to put them to use.

The Unpredictability of Multiple Sclerosis Offers Both Challenges and Opportunities

Life is unpredictable for all of us, but most of us aren't aware of, or in tune with, that unpredictability every day. People with MS, on the other hand, may experience that unpredictability from morning to night or day to day. While this is stressful and exhausting, it also offers you the opportunity to think about what matters to you now, in the moment. Is it rest, connecting with someone else, getting a task done, learning a new skill, getting in a bit of physical activity, providing help and support to another person, creating something beautiful—or something else entirely? Exploring your options, trying new things, or finding new ways to do familiar things all provide opportunities for growth, connection, and impact on the world around you. And in doing that kind of self-exploration and discovery, you find the things that continue to give your life meaning.

Finding Meaning Is Different from Understanding Why

One of the most common questions people ask following a diagnosis of MS, a worsening of symptoms, or a loss of cherished abilities, is "Why?" They want to know why this happened to them, what they did to cause it, or what they could have done to prevent it. They even ask what they did to deserve it. The scientific answers to these questions may provide some reassurance, but they don't acknowledge the feelings behind the "Why?" At this time, we do not know what causes MS or why one person develops it and another does not (see Chapter 1). However, we do know that MS likely results from a complex interaction of viral, environmental, and genetic factors. It is not a punishment, and it is *never* deserved. Difficult as it may be to accept, there is no clear reason behind it. The closest explanation may be lousy luck.

The good thing about lousy luck is that it levels the playing field. It can happen to anyone and it's up to you to find whatever meaning in it that allows you to step back, consider who you are and what's important to you, and then move forward with your life in ways that align with your values and priorities. If you feel frustrated or at a loss—unable to identify a path forward—working with a grief counselor or mental health professional can help you forge ahead.

We hope this book has helped you and your care partner(s) feel more informed, better prepared to manage MS and the symptoms that impact daily life, more confident in your ability to work collaboratively with the MS care team, and ready to nurture your wellness.

Multiple Sclerosis Disease-Modifying Therapies

Ask your provider for detailed information about the benefits, side effects, and risks of these medications, as well as information about the different ways in which they work in the body.

Route of Administration	Name	Dosing Frequency	Approval	Manufacturer's Support Services
Oral	Aubagio	Once daily	Relapsing forms of MS[a] in adults	None available through the drug manufacturer (1-855-676-6326)
	Bafiertam	Twice daily	Relapsing forms of MS in adults	https://www.bafiertam.com (1-855-322-6637)
	Dimethyl fumarate (generic equivalent of Tecfidera)	Twice daily	Relapsing forms of MS in adults	None available through the drug manufacturers
	Gilenya	Once daily	Relapsing forms of multiple sclerosis (MS), to include clinically isolated syndrome, relapsing-remitting disease, and active secondary progressive disease, in adults and children 10 years of age and older.	https://www.gilenya.com/c/ms-pill/go-program (1-800-445-3692)
	Mavenclad	Intermittent over 2 years	Relapsing–remitting MS and active secondary progressive MS in adults; generally recommended for those who did not respond to or were unable to tolerate other medications	https://www.mavenclad.com/en (1-877-447-3243)
	Mayzent	Once daily following start-up regimen	Relapsing forms of MS in adults	https://www.mayzent.com/financial-support (1-877-629-9368)
	Ponvory	Once daily following start-up regimen	Relapsing forms of MS in adults	https://ponvoryus.com/cost-and-savings

Route of Administration	Name	Dosing Frequency	Approval	Manufacturer's Support Services
	Tasenso ODT	Once daily	Relapsing forms of multiple sclerosis (MS), to include clinically isolated syndrome, relapsing-remitting disease, and active secondary progressive disease, in adults and children 10 years of age and older.	https://www.tascenso.com/patient/cycle-vita/hub-support
	Tecfdera	Twice daily	Relapsing forms of MS in adults	https://www.biogenoptions.com (1-800-456-2255)
	Vumerity	Twice daily	Relapsing forms of MS in adults	https://www.biogenoptions.com (1-800-456-2255)
	Zeposia	Once daily	Relapsing forms of MS in adults	https://www.zeposia.com (1-833-937-6742)
Self-injection	Avonex	Once daily	Relapsing forms of MS	https://www.biogenoptions.com (1-800-456-2255)
	Beta-eron	Every other day	Relapsing forms of MS in adults	https://www.patientassistance.bayer.us (1-844-788-1470)
	Copaxone	Daily or three times per week formulations	Relapsing forms of MS in adults	https://www.copaxone.com or https://www.mysharedsolutions.com (1-800-887-8100)

Route of Administration	Name	Dosing Frequency	Approval	Manufacturer's Support Services
	Glatopa (generic equivalent of Copaxone)	Daily or three times per week formulations	Relapsing forms of MS in adults	https://www.glatopa.com (1-855-452-8672)
	Glatiramer acetate injection (generic equivalent of Copaxone)	Daily or three times per week formulations	Relapsing forms of MS in adults	https://www.viatris.com/en-us/lm/united-states/patient-assistance-program
	Kesimpta	Every 4 weeks following a start-up regimen	Relapsing forms of MS in adults	https://www.kesimpta.com/patient-support/financial-resources (1-855-537-4678)
	Plegridy	Every 2 weeks following a start-up regimen	Relapsing forms of MS	https://www.biogenoptions.com (1-800-456-2255)
	Rebif	Three times per week	Relapsing forms of MS	https://www.mslifelines.com (1-877-447-3243)
Intravenous infusion	Briumvi	Every 24 weeks following start-up regimen	Relapsing forms of MS	https://www.briumvipatientsupport.com (1-833-274-8684)
	Lemtrada	First course: 5 consecutive days Second course 1 year later: 3 consecutive days	Relapsing–remitting MS and active secondary progressive MS in adults; generally recommended for those who had an inadequate response to two or more medications	https://www.lemtrada.com (1-855-676-6326)

Route of Administration	Name	Dosing Frequency	Approval	Manufacturer's Support Services
	Novantrone	Every 3 months	Worsening relapsing MS; secondary progressive MS; progressive relapsing MS in adults	None available through the drug manufacturer.
	Ocrevus	Every 6 months following a start-up regimen	Relapsing forms of MS as well as primary progressive MS in adults	https://www.genentech-access.com (1-877-436-3683)
	Tysabri	Every 4 weeks	To be used only as a monotherapy (not in combination with other DMTs) with relapsing forms of MS in adults	https://www.biogenoptions.com (1-800-456-2255)
	Tyruko	Every 4 weeks	To be used only as a monotherapy (not in combination with other DMTs) with relapsing forms of MS in adults	https://www.tyruko.com

[a]Relapsing forms of MS include clinically isolated syndrome, relapsing–remitting MS, and active secondary progressive MS. DMTs, disease-modifying therapies; MS, multiple sclerosis.

Additional Medication Financial Assistance Programs

Good Rx

https://www.GoodRx.com

For additional assistance, Phone: 1-855-268-282 or email: ada@goodrx.com

HealthWell Foundation

www.healthwellfoundation.org

Phone: (800) 675-8416

Patient Access Network (PAN) Foundation
www.panfoundation.org
Phone: (866) 316-7263

Patient Advocate Foundation (PAF)
www.patientadvocate.org
Phone: (866) 512-3861

Patient Help Network
https://www.patienthelpnetwork.org
1-866-828-7288

For additional prescription assistance resources, contact:

The National Multiple Sclerosis Society
https://www.Contact Us | National MS Society
Phone: 1-800-344-4867

Multiple Sclerosis Association of America
MSAA's Helpline: (800) 532-7667, ext. 154

Resources

Multiple Sclerosis Advocacy Organizations

Multiple Sclerosis Coalition—A collaborative network of independent multiple sclerosis organizations whose objectives are education, advocacy, collaboration, and the effective use of resources for the benefit of the entire multiple sclerosis (MS) community. The following are the member organizations:

1. **Accelerated Cure Project for Multiple Sclerosis**—The goal of the Accelerated Cure Project is to accelerate research toward a cure for MS by: involving people affected by MS in the entire research process, from the design of studies to the impact of results on their daily lives; create data and biosample resources for use by researchers worldwide; and promote the sharing of study results by all MS researchers as a way to optimize their impact.
   Phone: 1-781-487-0008
   https://www.acceleratedcure.org
2. **Can Do Multiple Sclerosis**—Can Do Multiple Sclerosis offers free educational and group coaching programs designed to help people living with MS (and care partners) achieve their personal health and wellness goals—physical, emotional,

cognitive, social, and spiritual (https://cando-ms.org/progr ams; https://cando-ms.org/?s=support+partner). The organization helps those affected by MS better understand the ways MS impacts their daily lives and learn how to increase their motivation to make healthful changes. Can Do Multiple Sclerosis offers a comprehensive online exercise program (https://www. cando-ms.org/exercises) as well as personalized guidance to overcome challenges while building social connections and a positive support network.

Phone: 1-800-367-3101

https://cando-ms.org

3. **The Consortium of Multiple Sclerosis Centers**—This is a nonprofit organization for health care professionals who work to improve the lives of all those affected by MS. The organization's mission is to develop and sustain successful models of care to address the MS disease spectrum; stimulate and facilitate MS research; develop mechanisms for sharing information with its members and all those affected by MS; and influence health care delivery in MS and related disorders.

Phone: 1-201-487-1050

https://www.mscare.org

4. **International Organization of Multiple Sclerosis Nurses**— This organization's mission is to establish and perpetuate a specialized branch of nursing in MS; establish standards of nursing care in MS; support MS nursing research; educate the health care community about MS; and disseminate this knowledge throughout the world.

Phone: 1-201-487-1050

https://iomsn.org

5. **Multiple Sclerosis Association of America**—This organization improves the lives of people affected by MS through vital services and support, including the provision of assistive devices such as grab bars, shower chairs, canes, walkers, and wheelchairs at no charge to individuals living with MS. It also

offers a comprehensive guide to disease-modifying therapies (https://mymsaa.org/ms-information/treatments/guide).

Phone: 1-800-532-7667

https://mymsaa.org

6. **Multiple Sclerosis Foundation**—The Multiple Sclerosis Foundation, known in the MS community as MS Focus, is a nonprofit organization focused on providing free services that address the critical needs of people with MS and their families, helping them maintain the best quality of life. The foundation provides grants (https://msfocus.org/Get-Help.aspx) for emergency assistance, exercise programming, homecare assistance, transportation assistance, and cooling apparel, among others.

Phone: 1-800-225-6495

https://msfocus.org

7. **MS Views and News**—MS Views and News is a patient advocacy organization that provides educational programs, advocacy, and resources to empower and enhance quality of life for the MS community.

Phone: 1-786-286-8777

https://msviewsandnews.org

8. **National Multiple Sclerosis Society**—The Society's research mission is to stop disease progression, restore lost function, and eradicate the disease. The Society's programs and services include MS Navigators, who provide information, resources, and support (https://www.nationalmssociety.org/Resources-Support); employment and financial planning resources (https://www.nationalmssociety.org/Living-Well-With-MS/Work-and-Home/Insurance-and-Financial-Information/Social-Security-Disability; healthcare providers and resources (https://www.nationalmssociety.org/Helpful-Links/Contact-Us/Find-Doctors and Other Resources), the Edward M. Dowd Personal Advocate Program, which connects people with advanced MS to intensive care management services; and an extensive array of free publications about all aspects of life

with MS (https://www.nationalmssociety.org/Resources-Supp ort/Library-Education-Programs).

Phone: 1-800-344-4867

https://www.nationalmssociety.org

9. **United Spinal Association**—United Spinal Association supports and advocates for the 5.5 million wheelchair users in the United States. It uses today's tools to directly provide services and resources to its members, chapters, and the broader disability community.

Fax: 1-718-803-3782

https://unitedspinal.org

Additional Resources

About Multiple Sclerosis

Your best online sources of information about MS are websites ending in .org or .edu, which are nonprofit or academic sites; websites ending in .com are commercial. In addition to the Multiple Sclerosis Coalition members listed above, consider also the following:

- MS Trust—https://mstrust.org.uk
  - A-to-Z of MS—https://mstrust.org.uk/a-z
- National Institutes of Health—https://www.ninds.nih.gov
  - MS information—https://www.ninds.nih.gov/health-info rmation/disorders/multiple-sclerosis
- Healthline—https://www.healthline.com

Who Gets Multiple Sclerosis

- "Racial and Ethnic Disparities in Multiple Sclerosis Prevalence"—https://www.neurology.org/content/98/18/e1818

- "Population-Based Estimates for the Prevalence of Multiple Sclerosis in the United States by Race, Ethnicity, Age, Sex, and Geographic Region"—https://www.ncbi.nlm.nih.gov/pmc/artic les/PMC10186207
- "Kids Get MS Too: A Guide for Parents of a Child or Teen with MS"
- "Kids Get MS Too: A Guide for Parents of a Child or Teen with MS"—https://www.msif.org/resource/a-guide-for-pare nts-of-a-child-or-teen-with-ms/

Help with Your Mental Health

- Mental Health America (https://mhanational.org)—a community-based nonprofit that promotes mental health through advocacy, education, research, and services
  - Where to get help—https://www.mhanational.org/im-look ing-mental-health-help-myself
  - Free, online, confidential screening tools for depression, anxiety, and other mental health issues—https://screening. mhanational.org
  - Mental health wellness tools—https://mhanational.org/b4sta ge4-get-help
- *Psychology Today*, "Find a Therapist"—https://www.psycholo gytoday.com/us
- Online Therapy directory—https://www.onlinetherapy.com
- National Institutes of Health, "Help for Mental Illnesses"— https://www.nimh.nih.gov/health/find-help
- Free access article: "Recommendations for Cognitive Screening and Management in Multiple Sclerosis Care"—https://doi.org/ 10.1177/1352458518803785

Intimacy and Sexuality

- (Book) *The Guide to Getting It On*, by Paul Joannides, PsyD
- (Book) *Come as You Are*, by Emily Nagoski, PhD

Support for Support Partners

- The MS Care Partner Connection—https://mscarepartnercon nection.com
- For questions/feedback and suggestions—https://mscarepartne rconnection.com/contact-us
- National Family Caregivers Association—https://caringco mmunity.org
- Family Caregiver Alliance—https://www.caregiver.org
- Caregiver Action Network—https://www.caregiveraction.org

Health and Wellness

- Free access article: "Exercise and Lifestyle Physical Activity Recommendations for People with Multiple Sclerosis Throughout the Disease Course"—https://doi.org/10.1177/ 1352458520915629
- (Book) *Optimal Health with Multiple Sclerosis: A Guide to Integrating Lifestyle, Alternative, and Conventional Medicine*, by Allen Bowling, MD, PhD

Employment

- Job Accommodation Network—https://askjan.org: a source of free, expert, and confidential guidance on job accommodations and disability employment issues, including one-on-one practical guidance and technical assistance on job accommodation solutions to help a person stay in the workforce

Staying Up-to-Date with Multiple Sclerosis Research

- *Multiple Sclerosis News Today*—https://multiplesclerosisnewsto
day.com

Participate in Multiple Sclerosis Research

- National Institutes of Health—https://clinicaltrials.gov
- The Accelerated Cure Project for Multiple Sclerosis—www.
acceleratedcure.org

Disease-Modifying Therapy Financial Support Programs

- See Appendix 1

GLOSSARY

abducens nerve: the nerve that allows the eye to look side to side.

acute disseminated encephalomyelitis: an acute, rapidly progressive autoimmune process that causes demyelination in the brain and spinal cord. It results from inflammation that occurs in response to a viral or bacterial infection or, less commonly, to an immunization.

advocacy organizations: Multiple sclerosis (MS) advocacy organizations provide information, emotional support, and connection opportunities for individuals living with MS; advocate at all levels of government on behalf of people affected by MS; and raise funds to support research and services.

ageusia: the complete loss of taste—an uncommon but possible symptom of MS.

anemia: a condition caused by insufficient numbers of healthy red blood cells, which leads to reduced oxygen flow to the body's organs.

ankle dorsiflexors: muscles that allow the ankle to flex upward during walking so that the toes clear the ground. Weakened dorsiflexors result in "foot drop" and other gait changes.

ankle–foot orthotic (AFO): an L-shaped plastic or lightweight carbon fiber device that fits under the foot and up the back of the weak leg to prevent the foot from "dropping" forward.

anosmia: the loss of the sense of smell—an uncommon but possible symptom of MS.

antigen: any substance (e.g., toxin, virus, bacteria, or chemical) that provokes an immune response against the substance. In MS, this is likely a protein that provokes the immune system to attack cells and tissues in the CNS.

anxiety: a symptom of MS as well as a reaction to the challenges of a chronic, unpredictable illness. Anxiety, which can range from mild to severe, is characterized by intense and persistent worry about everyday events, as well as physical symptoms such as rapid heart rate, rapid breathing, and other physical changes.

ataxia: a significant loss of muscle control that causes clumsy movement or speech. It can occur in the limbs, the trunk, with walking, or with speech.

atrophy: the progressive degeneration of tissue. In MS, atrophy can occur in muscles due to disuse or in the brain due to demyelination and destruction of nerve cells.

autoimmune disease: a disease in which the body's immune system mistakenly attacks and damages healthy cells.

autonomic nervous system: the "control system" that governs the body's reflexive, automatic functions—things that happen without conscious thought, such as heart rate, digestion, respiration rate, salivation, and perspiration.

axon: the wire-like extension of the neuron that sends messages from one part of the brain to another.

Babinski sign: an abnormal reflex response, often seen in MS, that signals damaged nerve pathways. The normal reflex causes the toes to point downward when the sole of the foot is stroked with a blunt instrument. When the reflex is abnormal, the big toe points upward and the toes fan outwards.

baclofen pump: a surgically implanted pump, used to treat severe spasticity, that delivers baclofen directly into the spinal canal through a tube.

biomarker: any substance, structure, or process that can be measured in the body, or in bodily products, which indicates the presence of disease, disease changes, or responses to treatment.

blood–brain barrier: highly selective, semipermeable blood vessels that form a barrier between the circulating blood and the brain, allowing some necessary cells and substances into the brain but restricting other cells and substances that could be harmful.

body mapping exercise: an activity that allows a person to learn what parts of their body feel good and have pleasurable sensations when touched. By periodically spending time alone to explore their own body and learn what feels good and what doesn't, the person is better able to teach their sexual partner what has changed (due to MS, normal aging, or other factors), what feels the same, and what would feel most pleasurable.

cacosmia: a disordered sense of smell that causes normal smells to be foul or stinking—an uncommon but possible symptom of MS.

caregiver: a care partner who also provides hands-on care or assistance on an ongoing basis.

care partner: any family member or friend who provides support and assistance on an ongoing basis to a person with a disease or condition (in this case, MS). Also referred to as a "support partner."

central nervous system (CNS): composed of the brain and spinal cord and optic nerve, the CNS coordinates the activity of all parts of the body.

central vein sign: a finding on magnetic resonance imaging (MRI) that is considered a marker for MS. It shows a vein within a white matter lesion.

cerebrospinal: referring to the brain (cerebro) and the spine (spinal).

cerebrospinal fluid (CSF): a clear, watery fluid formed by the tissues in the ventricles (hollow structures) within the brain that flows around the surface of the brain and spinal cord. Its functions are to protect the brain and spinal cord from injury, provide nutrients, and remove waste.

cervical: refers to the area of the spine at the neck, including vertebrae 1–7.

clinically isolated syndrome (CIS): a first episode of a clinical symptom or symptoms caused by an abnormality in the brain or spinal cord that is consistent with CNS inflammation but does meet the diagnostic criteria for MS.

cognitive–behavioral therapy: a form of talk therapy that helps a person become aware of inaccurate or negative thinking that interferes with their ability to function in daily life, in their relationships, and in challenging situations at home or work. It is generally structured and short term, and it is effective in treating depression and other mood problems, as well as sleep disorders and even symptoms of MS including pain and fatigue.

cognitive dysfunction: a common symptom of MS that may include problems with information processing, memory, attention, word-finding during conversations, visuospatial skills, and/or complex processes such as planning, prioritizing, organizing, decision-making, and judgment.

cognitive fatigue: a debilitating mental exhaustion that a person can experience during a cognitively demanding task which requires intense focus or concentration. Often described as "hitting a wall," this type of fatigue forces a person to stop the task and rest and relax their mind before resuming the task.

cognitive remediation: treatment strategies to help people improve their cognitive function in everyday life. The remediation sessions typically consist of computerized exercise to improve attention and memory and personalized tools and strategies to help people compensate for problems with organization, decision-making, task completion, communication, and other life activities.

cognitive screening: a very brief assessment of cognitive function—most often a test of information processing speed—that is recommended for people with MS at the time of diagnosis and every 6–12 months thereafter. A positive screen indicates the need for a more in-depth cognitive evaluation.

cognitive specialist: a health care professional who assesses, diagnoses, and provides cognitive remediation for cognitive difficulties. The primary providers of these services include neuropsychologists, psychologists, speech–language pathologists, and occupational therapists.

color vision: the ability to see colors clearly, which may be disturbed or lost in a person with MS due to optic neuritis. With optic neuritis, colors may appear washed out, particularly reds, which may appear grayish.

comorbidity: an additional disease or medical condition that is not a complication of the first disease. When a person with MS has other conditions, such as depression, diabetes, heart disease, or another autoimmune condition, the non-MS conditions are referred to as comorbid conditions.

comprehensive MS care: includes disease management, symptom management (physical, emotional, and cognitive), rehabilitation, and attention to overall health and well-being.

contrast agent: a substance used to enhance the contrast of structures in medical imaging. In MS, gadolinium is used during some MRIs to highlight new or active lesions in the brain.

corticosteroid: a type of anti-inflammatory medicine that may be used in MS to speed recovery from a relapse. While often referred to as "steroids," they are distinct from the steroids used by some athletes to build muscle.

cranial nerves: twelve pairs of nerves that originate in the brain or brain stem and that control specific sensory and motor functions, particularly those involving the eyes, ears, nose, mouth, throat, face, and neck.

cytokines: small proteins that signal the cells of the immune system to defend us from viruses, bacteria, fungi, and parasites. Some cytokines are considered pro-inflammatory, which means they increase inflammation, whereas others are considered anti-inflammatory, which means they stop inflammation.

deconditioning: weakening of muscles due to disuse.

deep tendon reflexes: five reflexes that are evaluated during a standard neurologic exam: biceps, brachioradialis, triceps, patellar, and ankle. Some people with MS may have brisk or exaggerated reflexes (hyperreflexia), particularly early in the disease.

demyelination: the loss of the protective myelin coating around nerve fibers in the CNS caused by the inflammatory attack.

depression: a common symptom of MS as well as a reaction to the stresses of life with a chronic, unpredictable illness. Depression, which is characterized by persistent sadness and lack of interest in previously rewarding and pleasurable activities, can range from mild to severe.

detrusor muscle: the smooth muscle fibers that make up the bladder wall. The main purposes of the detrusor are to contract and push urine out into the urethra and to allow the bladder to stretch as urine accumulates.

detrusor–sphincter dyssynergia (DSD): occurs when the sphincter muscle or the urethra and the bladder (detrusor) muscle work against each other rather than in a coordinated way. The urethral sphincter fails to relax to allow urine to flow when the bladder contracts to release it, contributing to urinary symptoms.

detruser overactivity: increased or involuntary muscle contractions of the detrusor muscle of the bladder, resulting in bladder urgency, frequency, and incontinence.

diagnostic criteria: rules created by a team of MS and MRI experts for making an accurate and timely diagnosis of MS. The criteria have been revised over time based on advances in MRI technology and an evolving understanding of the MS disease process. The most current version of the criteria—the 2017 McDonald criteria—incorporates the neurologic examination, MRI findings, and spinal fluid analysis.

dietician: a highly trained and credentialed health care professional who counsels people on nutrition issues and healthy eating habits and can diagnose and treat certain types of food and diet-related conditions.

diplopia: double vision—or seeing double images—which occurs in MS when one of the three pairs of nerves that control eye movements is not working properly.

disability: a physical or mental condition that limits a person's movements, senses, or activities.

discriminative sense: the ability to feel the shape, size, texture, weight, and dimensionality of an object; the awareness of body parts and limb movements; the ability to sense vibration from a tuning fork. These senses are evaluated as part of the neurologic exam.

disease-modifying therapy (DMT): medication approved by regulatory agencies in the United States and other countries to treat the MS disease process. DMTs have been proven through clinical research to limit new symptoms, relapses, and inflammation in the CNS and delay disease progression.

dizziness: a term that describes feeling faint, woozy or unsteady. It can also be the sensation that the person feels that they or their surroundings are spinning which is termed vertigo.

dysesthesia: a distorted and painful sensation, such as burning or stabbing pain, that results from damage to nerves carrying sensory messages, which can occur anywhere in the body.

dysgeusia: an unpleasant taste sensation—an uncommon but possible symptom in MS.

dysmetria: Impaired ability to control the speed, distance, or range of physical movement. Dysmetria can produce the undershooting and overshooting of the intended movement toward a target.

epidemiologic studies: studies of how diseases behave in different populations and different locations.

Epstein–Barr virus (EBV): one of the most common viruses in people. EBV, which is in the herpes family, is the virus that causes mononucleosis. EBV remains in the body after exposure and has been shown to play a key role in the risk of developing MS.

evoked potential: a diagnostic test of the nerve pathways from the vision, hearing, or sensation pathways to the brain; also called an "evoked response."

evoked response: a diagnostic test of the nerve pathways from the vision, hearing, or sensation pathways to the brain; also called an "evoked potential."

exacerbation (also referred to as an attack, relapse, or flare): a neurologic symptom or symptoms that last a minimum of 24 hours and cannot be explained by any other cause, such as an elevated body temperature. The symptoms remain for a period of weeks to months and then completely or partially resolve.

executive function: a set of mental processes that helps connect past experience with present action; important for decision-making, judgment, planning, and organizing.

extensor tone: the amount of resistance to passive stretch when a limb is straightened. During the neurologic exam, the examiner assesses extensor tone by straightening the person's legs or arms.

foot drop: gait abnormality characterized by limited or no ability to lift the front of the foot.

forearm crutch (also called a Canadian or Lofstrand crutch): a crutch that has a cuff which goes around the forearm as well as a handle for the hand to grip. This kind of crutch offers greater comfort and stability than a standard crutch, particularly when used long term.

fundus: the inside, back surface of the eye that is made up of the retina, macula, optic disc, fovea, and blood vessels.

gadolinium: a contrast agent (injected into a vein) that can be used during an MRI to help identify abnormal tissue. In MS, it is used to identify areas of new inflammation.

gait: a person's manner of walking.

gene: the basic physical and functional unit of heredity passed from parent to child. Humans have between 20,000 and 25,000 genes, and each gene carries instructions to tell the cells in our body how to work. More than 200 gene variations have been found to contribute to a person's risk of developing MS.

genetic: related to gene activity.

glucocorticoid: a type of corticosteroid that has anti-inflammatory properties and is used to treat MS relapses. Glucocorticoids help speed recovery from a relapse but do not impact long-term disease outcomes.

gray matter: the unmyelinated areas of the brain and spinal cord that consist largely of neuronal cell bodies. The cells of gray matter allow us to process information.

gut–brain axis: the interactions between the immune system, nervous system, and the gut.

gut microbiota: the organisms that live in the human gut (gut flora), including bacteria, fungi, parasites, and viruses, among others, which play a critical role in our development, immune functions, and the digestion of the foods we eat. Each person's gut biota is unique, influenced by a variety of factors, including the foods they eat.

health coach: an expert in behavior change who guides clients who are seeking to make positive lifestyle shifts such as quitting smoking, eating a healthier diet, or becoming more physically active.

health psychologist: a psychologist who specializes in the biological, social, and psychological factors that influence health and illness.

high-efficacy DMT: an MS DMT that is considered to be more powerful and effective in reducing inflammation and disease activity. Currently, the DMTs considered to be higher efficacy (with greater associated risks) are alemtuzumab, cladribine, fingolimod, natalizumab, ocrelizumab, siponimod, ozanimod, and ofatumumab.

hip flexion assist device: a device designed to improve gait in individuals who have difficulty initiating the leg swing because of weakness in the hip flexor muscle.

hip flexor: the muscle that works to raise the knee toward the chest.

immune system: a system of cells, chemicals, biological structures, and processes that protects against disease by attacking foreign "intruders," such as viruses, bacteria, parasites, and cancer cells.

incontinence: involuntary loss of urine or stool.

inflammation: a carefully orchestrated response of the immune system to threats such as injury, irritation, or infection or in diseases such as multiple sclerosis.

information processing: the way the brain acquires, records, organizes, and uses the data coming in through the senses of vision, hearing, taste, touch, and smell. Slowed processing of information is the hallmark of cognitive difficulties in people with MS.

insomnia: difficulty with falling asleep or staying asleep.

intermittent self-catheterization: a strategy for emptying your bladder when you have difficulty urinating or emptying your bladder completely on your own. You insert a thin, hollow tube (catheter) into the bladder through the urethra to allow the urine to drain out of your bladder into the toilet, and then you remove the catheter. This may be done one or more times a day, as needed.

intravenous immunoglobulin (IVIG): a preparation of antibodies (immune globulin) obtained from pooled human blood samples, which are injected back into the body through a vein over the course of several days to help improve immune function. It has been used to help prevent a postpartum relapse and may also be used in people who are unable to tolerate or who have not had benefit from other relapse treatments.

irritability: feeling impatient, quick-tempered, hypersensitive, or reactive. Irritability, which is commonly reported by people with MS, can be a symptom of depression.

lassitude: an overwhelming sense of tiredness that materializes without warning or cause. It is not necessarily associated with exertion or heat exposure, but in some instances it can be exacerbated by factors such as heat, stress, sleep disruption, or medications.

lateral ventricles: paired structures with projections called "horns" into the frontal, temporal, and occipital lobes of the brain.

lesion: a general term that refers to damage or an abnormality in any body tissue or organ such as an injury. In multiple sclerosis, abnormal areas from inflammation or damage, which are visualized on MRI, are often referred to as lesions (see also *plaque*).

Lhermitte's sign: A buzzing, vibrating, or tingling sensation that goes down the back or into the body when the neck is flexed forward. This suggests the presence of nerve damage in the cervical (neck) portion of the spinal cord.

libido: sex drive or desire for sex.

licensed professional counselor: a mental health professional who offers mental health and substance abuse services.

lifestyle factors: the modifiable habits and ways of life (e.g., diet, exercise, sleep habits, smoking, and substance use) that can greatly influence overall health and wellness.

lifestyle modification: refers to the changes that people choose to make in their lifestyle in order to improve their health and wellness, such as quitting smoking, increasing their exercise, or opting for a healthier diet.

lifestyle physical activity: all planned or unplanned moderate to vigorous activities (leisure, household, or occupational) in a person's day.

Lofstrand crutch   (also known as a forearm crutch or Canadian crutch): This crutch has a forearm cuff and handgrip that are designed to provide stability and comfort.

lumbar puncture (spinal tap): the procedure of taking a small amount of fluid from the space around the spinal cord in the lower back through a hollow needle, usually done for diagnostic purposes. In MS, spinal fluid may show evidence of abnormal immune system activity.

magnetic resonance imaging (MRI): an imaging tool that uses a magnetic field and radio waves (rather than radiation) to create detailed images of the organs and tissues within the body.

major depression: a mental health disorder characterized by persistent low mood and/or disinterest in life activities, which causes a significant disruption in daily life. Major depressive episodes are a symptom of MS, but genetics, life challenges, and other factors are contributing factors.

McDonald criteria: a set of rules used by health care providers to ensure that they can diagnose MS as early and accurately as possible. The first set of criteria, developed by Ian McDonald in 2001, has been revised several times as MRI technology has become more advanced and our understanding of the MS disease process has grown.

mental health screening: brief tests that can identify possible depression, anxiety, or other mental disorders. A positive screen would suggest that a more comprehensive evaluation is needed in order to identify the appropriate treatment.

migraine: a common relapsing–remitting neurologic disease, sometimes misdiagnosed as MS, that causes a variety of symptoms, including pulsing headaches on one side of the head and, in some individuals, a group of sensory, motor, or speech symptoms called an aura.

mobility aide: any tool that is manufactured or adapted to assist a person to perform a particular task. Mobility aids, which include canes, walkers, rollators, crutches, wheelchairs, and orthotic devices such as braces or ankle–foot orthoses, help people remain safe and independent in their daily activities.

mononucleosis: a disease caused by EBV that spreads through saliva. Most adults have been exposed to EBV and have built up antibodies to it.

motorized scooter: a three- or four-wheeled, battery-powered mobility aid with a seat, steering mechanism, and brakes that allows people to conserve energy as they move from place to place.

MS care provider: the health care provider who collaborates with you to manage your MS. Neurologists, as well as advance practice providers (nurse practitioners and physician assistants), provide this type of ongoing neurologic care.

MS fatigue (also known as lassitude): the most common and often the most disabling symptom of MS. Its exact cause is unknown, but it generally occurs daily; tends to worsen over the course of the day; and may be worsened by heat, humidity, or cold.

MS hug: a symptom of MS that feels like an uncomfortable, even painful, feeling of tightness around the stomach or chest.

multiple sclerosis (MS): a chronic disease that affects the body's CNS, or brain and spinal cord, and commonly produces symptoms that can include fatigue, numbness, weakness, stiffness, bowel and bladder difficulties, vision change, and loss of balance, among others.

muscle tone: how loose or stiff the muscles are.

musculoskeletal pain (also called orthopedic pain): may occur in MS due to changes in a person's gait, use of an inappropriate mobility aid, incorrect use of the aid, muscle strain, changes in posture, or inactivity.

myelin: an insulating layer composed of proteins and fats that surrounds most nerve fibers; it both protects the nerve fibers and accelerates nerve impulse transmission.

myelin oligodendrocyte glycoprotein antibody-associated disease (MOGAD): a neuroinflammatory condition that most often causes inflammation in the optic nerve but can also cause inflammation in the spinal cord and brain. Myelin oligodendrocyte glycoprotein, a protein on the surface of myelin sheaths, is an immune target in this disease.

nerve cells: the core components of the nervous system, which process and transmit information to and from the brain and spinal cord based on electrical and chemical signaling.

nerve fiber (also known as axon): a wire-like extension of the neuron that sends messages from one part of the brain to another.

nerve fiber fatigue: temporary weakness, visual loss, or cognitive changes that are provoked by sustained activity or heat exposure.

nerve growth factors: proteins that help develop and maintain nerve cells.

nerve impulses: waves of chemical and electrical excitement that travel along nerve fibers in response to a stimulus.

neurodegeneration: a slow and progressive loss of nerve cells in the brain due to inflammation and damage over time. It is associated with progressive physical and cognitive disability.

neurofilament light chain(NfL) a member of the intermediate filament protein family, which is being studied as a biomarker of MS disease activity and neuronal damage in the CNS.

neurologic exam: an evaluation of a person's nervous system. The exam includes assessment of motor and sensory functions, balance and coordination, mental status, reflexes, and nerve function.

neurologist: a medical doctor and specialist in the nervous system and the disorders affecting it.

neurology: the branch of medicine that deals with the diagnosis and treatment of nervous system disorders.

neuromyelitis optica spectrum disorder (NMOSD): a rare relapsing autoimmune disorder that most often causes inflammation in the optic nerve and spinal cord. Although once considered a variant of MS, it is differentiated from MS by a different disease process in the body, more severe attacks, and different targets in the CNS.

neuropathic pain: pain that is caused by damage or inflammation in the brain or spinal cord. The nerve damage might cause a range of sensations, from minor irritations to intense stabbing, burning, or squeezing sensations.

neuropsychologist: an expert in how brain injuries and diseases can affect a person's behavior, mood, and thinking skills. In MS, neuropsychologists evaluate mood and cognitive function and provide cognitive rehabilitation.

neurotransmitters: chemical messengers that allow cells of the nervous system to communicate with one another.

nocturia: waking up more than once during the night to urinate.

nocturnal spasm: involuntary muscle contractions that occur during the night, which are caused by spasticity. They can be extremely painful and disrupt sleep.

numbness: a complete or partial loss of feeling or sensation in an area of the body.

nurse practitioner (NP): a nurse with advanced clinical education and training who performs physical exams, makes diagnoses, treats diseases, and prescribes medications. Many NPs specialize in the diagnosis and treatment of MS in neurology offices and comprehensive MS care centers.

nutritionist: a person who advises others about ways that food and nutrition impact their health. Many nutritionists have advanced degrees and many states require licensure for nutritionists to practice. However, the term nutritionist is not regulated in every state.

nystagmus: involuntary eye movement that causes the eye to move rapidly from side to side, up and down, or in a circle.

occipital nerve: transmits sensation to the skin from the back of the scalp to the top of the head.

occipital neuralgia: inflammation of the occipital nerves, which causes severe piercing, throbbing, or shock-like pain in the upper neck, back of the head, or behind the ears.

occupational therapy: therapy that focuses on the performance of daily activities, with attention to energy management, environmental modifications, task simplification, and adaptive tools for home and work.

oculomotor nerve: helps to adjust and coordinate eye position during movement.

off-label: a term that describes the use of a medication in ways other than what it was approved for by the U.S. Food and Drug Administration (FDA). Once a medication has been FDA-approved, a licensed physician can choose to prescribe it for other purposes.

oligoclonal bands: certain immune proteins that appear in the cerebrospinal fluid and indicate abnormal immune activity. Most people with MS have evidence of oligoclonal bands in their cerebrospinal fluid, making it an important finding in the MS diagnostic process.

oligodendrocytes: the myelin-forming cells in the CNS.

ophthalmologist: a medical doctor specializing in eye and vision care who can diagnose and treat a wide range of conditions, perform surgery, and prescribe glasses and contact lenses. MS may be initially recognized by an ophthalmologist who detects inflammatory damage to the optic nerve during an eye exam.

ophthalmoscope: an instrument used to look at the back of the eye.

optical coherence tomography (OCT): OCT is a noninvasive imaging test that used light waves to take pictures of the retina. In MS, OCT is used to measure the nerve fiber layer of the retina in the eye, which correlates with nerve damage (neurodegeneration) in the CNS.

optic nerve: the nerve in each eye that transmits visual information from the retina to the brain.

optic neuritis: inflammation of the optic nerve causing vision impairment in one eye.

orthotist: a health care professional who designs and makes customized supportive devises such as a leg brace or ankle–foot orthosis to assist people with their mobility.

paresthesia: an abnormal sensation—typically numbness, tingling, or prickling—caused by damage to nerves carrying sensory messages.

pathology: the study of disease and the changes in body tissues and organs that cause or are caused by disease.

pelvic floor physical therapy: a treatment that addresses dysfunction in the muscles of the pelvic floor that support the urinary and reproductive tracts.

percutaneous tibial nerve stimulation(PTNS): a nonsurgical office procedure that provides electrical stimulation to the tibial nerve in the lower leg that is responsible for bladder control. It is used in the treatment of urinary urgency, frequency, and incontinence.

periodic plateaus: periods when the disease is stable.

peripheral nervous system (PNS): extends throughout the body and is responsible for connecting the CNS to the limbs and organs.

physical activity: a general term that applies to all activities a person engages in, including lifestyle physical activities (e.g., bathing, dressing, walking, cleaning, or mowing the lawn), and structured exercise that is done repeatedly to improve a function, such as strength, endurance, balance, or flexibility.

physical therapist (PT): a rehabilitation professional who focuses on mobility, strength, flexibility, balance, and pain management, with the goal of improving or maintaining function, safety, and independence. PTs who specialize in MS care are often certified as neurologic clinical specialists.

physical therapy: interventions by trained professionals to assess and treat problems with mobility (walking, balance, spasticity, and falls) and musculoskeletal pain.

physician assistant (PA): a licensed advanced practice clinician who is trained to diagnose and treat patients, perform medical procedures, prescribe medications, order tests, and develop treatment plans. Many PAs work in neurology practices or MS comprehensive care centers to treat MS patients.

plaque: scar tissue in the CNS that forms when the MS immune attack causes damage to the myelin that surrounds the nerve fibers. Plaques are evidence of demyelination. This scarring—or *sclerosis*—is what gives the disease its name.

plasma: the liquid portion of blood that carries the blood cells.

plasmapheresis (also called plasma exchange or PLEX): a therapeutic intervention that involves removing plasma containing harmful antibodies from a person's blood and replacing it with healthy fluid. In MS, PLEX is sometimes used to treat severe relapses that do not respond to treatment with corticosteroids.

polyunsaturated fatty acids (PUFAs): the omega-3 and omega-6 fats that are essential to health brain function. PUFAs, which are liquid at room temperature, must be obtained from the foods we eat.

position sense: awareness of where body parts are in relation to one another and where the body is in space.

preventive health screening: health care services such as tests or screenings that are performed to check a person's health status and identify conditions that may need treatment. Examples include blood pressure, diabetes, and cholesterol tests, as well as cancer screenings such as mammograms, prostate-specific antigen (PSA) testing for prostate cancer, and colonoscopies. Preventive health screening is particularly important for people with MS, who may have comorbid health conditions that can speed the progression of their disease.

primary MS fatigue: the sense of feeling tired physically and/or cognitively, that results directly from the MS disease process.

primary progressive MS (PPMS): an MS disease course marked by a slow decline in neurologic function from the start, which may plateau at times but has no sharply identifiable relapses or remissions.

primary sexual problems: changes in sexual feelings and responses caused directly by damage in the CNS. In men and women, this may include decreased interest; reduced arousal (e.g., problems with vaginal lubrication or erections); difficulty achieving orgasm; and sensory changes such as numbness, tingling, or pain that interfere with sexual activity.

progression: continued disease activity, independent of relapses, that is often associated with accumulation of disability. The acronym PIRA (progression independent of relapses) is often used to describe progression that is not associated with a relapse.

progressive MS: a term used to describe two MS disease courses: primary progressive MS(PPMS), which is progressive from onset with few or new relapses, and secondary progressive MS(SPMS), which follows an initial relapsing–remitting disease course. In general, progressive MS is characterized by gradual disease worsening and nerve damage, whereas relapsing MS is characterized more by inflammation.

proprioception: awareness of the position of one's body in space.

pseudoexacerbation (pseudorelapse): an acute aggravation of an existing symptom caused by overexertion or elevation in body temperature due to an infection or hot, humid weather. Exposure to cold can also cause a pseudoexacerbation in some people.

psychiatrist: a medical doctor who specializes in the diagnosis and treatment of mental disorders, with a focus on medication management.

psychologist: a mental health professional who uses a variety of therapeutic techniques to help people process personal and family issues; diagnose and treat depression, anxiety, and other mood disorders; and manage cognitive challenges. They may offer individual, group, and/or family therapy.

radiologically isolated syndrome (RIS): evidence of neurologic damage, consistent with MS, that is found incidentally in a person receiving an MRI of the brain for a medical condition other than MS (e.g., head injury or migraines). Approximately 50% of people with RIS go on to develop clinical features of MS within 10 years.

radiologist: a medical doctor who specializes in diagnosing and treating diseases using medical imaging tests such as X-rays, computed tomography (CT) scans, or MRI scans. In MS, the radiologist and the MS care provider assess MRI scans for signs of inflammatory damage in the CNS.

rebound relapses: when a person who has discontinued treatment with certain DMTs abruptly experiences new disease activity.

reflex: an unconscious reaction to a stimulus. In MS, certain reflexes, known as deep tendon reflexes, are abnormal and tend to be overactive. One example in MS is the knee-jerk response that occurs when a provider taps the knee with a reflex hammer.

rehabilitation: a type of care that helps a person regain, retain, or improve function in everyday life.

rehabilitation specialist: a provider (physical therapist, occupational therapist, speech–language pathologist, or physiatrist) who focuses on helping a person recover, retain, or improve functioning following a change in abilities.

relapse (also referred to as an attack, exacerbation, or flare): a neurologic symptom or symptoms that last a minimum of 24 hours and cannot be explained by any other cause. The symptoms remain for a period of weeks to months and then completely or partially resolve.

relapse-associated worsening (RAW): incomplete recovery from a relapse with persistent symptoms that may cause disability.

relapsing forms of MS: clinically isolated syndrome, relapsing–remitting MS, and active secondary progressive MS (with relapses or evidence of new lesions on MRI along with disease progression).

relapsing–remitting MS (RRMS): the most common MS disease type, which is characterized by clearly defined attacks (also called relapses or exacerbations) of new or worsening neurologic symptoms that are followed by periods of partial or complete recovery. RRMS can also be characterized as either *active* (with relapses or evidence of new activity on MRI) or *not active*, as well as *worsening* (with a confirmed increase in disability following a relapse) or *not worsening.*

remission: a period of partial or complete recovery following an MS exacerbation.

residual symptoms: the symptoms that remain when recovery from a relapse is less than 100%.

restless leg syndrome: unpleasant tickling or twitching sensation in the leg muscles when sitting or lying down, which is relieved only by moving the legs.

rollator: a mobility aid that is sometimes called a "wheeled" walker. A rollator consists of a frame with three or four large wheels, handlebars, and a built-in seat that allows for rest during a walk. Because they come in a wide range of styles, it is helpful to work with a physical therapist when searching for the rollator that best meets your needs.

S1P receptor modulators: a class of MS DMT that prevents white blood cells (lymphocytes) from leaving the lymph nodes, which reduces the number of lymphocytes that can enter the CNS.

saturated fats: fats, including butter, lard, animal fats, and some fats from plants, that are solid at room temperature and are thought to contribute to inflammation.

scissoring gait: a walking pattern characterized by knees and thighs pressured together or crossing each other. In MS, a scissoring gait can be caused by abnormal muscle tone or spasticity.

sclerosis: a hardening of tissue, often from an overgrowth of fibrous tissue.

seating and mobility specialist (SMS): certified assistive technology professionals who assess a person's mobility needs; recommend the appropriate wheeled mobility aid(s); and ensure that the equipment offers the optimal support, comfort, and utility for each individual.

secondary MS fatigue: the sense of feeling tired that is provoked by a non-MS source, such as another illness, depression, stress, medication side effects, poor sleep, or overexertion.

secondary progressive MS (SPMS): a disease course that often follows relapsing–remitting MS and is characterized by disease worsening over time and may include periods of stability and occasional relapses, especially early in the disease course.

secondary sexual problems: changes in sexual interest or activity resulting from other symptoms of MS, such as fatigue, spasticity, pain, and bladder problems, or from side effects of medications that increase fatigue or vaginal dryness.

sensation: the ability to feel physical stimuli such as heat, cold, pain, or pressure.

sensory ataxia: unsteady walking, standing, or other movements due to disruption in the spinal cord or brain that interferes with the nerves carrying information about the position of the body and/or limbs.

sensory symptoms: include problems with vision, distorted sensations or pain, and loss of feeling. Changes in the senses—hearing, taste, smell—can also occur.

separation in space: refers to the criteria for diagnosing MS, which state that there must be evidence that the initial episodes of neuronal damage occurred in different places in the CNS.

separation in time: refers to the criteria for diagnosing MS, which state that there must be evidence that the initial episodes of neuronal damage occurred at distinct points in time.

sepsis: a life-threatening complication of an existing infection any-where in the body. It occurs when chemicals released into the bloodstream cause a series of changes that damage multiple organ systems, potentially leading to organ failure and some-times death.

sex chromosomes: The genetic material on X and Y chromosomes that determines biologic sexual characteristics.

sex hormones: proteins produced by the ovaries and testicles that help determine sexual function and characteristics. They can also act on the immune and nervous systems.

shared decision-making: a process in which health care providers and people with MS work together to make decisions about treatments, tests, and management strategies. These decisions are based on both the person's preferences, goals, and values and clinical evidence, in-cluding risks and benefits.

short-chain fatty acids: compounds produced from certain foods by the gut biome, which are thought to have anti-inflammatory properties.

sleep apnea: periods of disrupted breathing during sleep, which interfere with restful sleep in many people with MS.

sleep specialist: a health care professional (physician, psycholo-gist, psychiatrist, among others) who diagnoses and treats sleep disturbances and disorders. They conduct thorough sleep assessments and offer treatment for insomnia, sleep apnea, restless leg syndrome, circadian rhythm disorders, and several types of ab-normal sleep behavior.

smoldering MS: a term used to describe ongoing MS disease activity in the CNS independent of relapses, which may explain why some people feel worse yet have no evidence of new disease activity (relapses or new MRI lesions).

Social Security disability (SSD): a tax-funded federal insurance program (Society Security Disability Insurance [SSDI]) in the United States that is managed by the Social Security Administration. It provides monthly benefits to people who have a disability that restricts their ability to work. Another program, called Supplemental Security Income(SSI) provides basic financial assistance to people with disabilities who have been unable to work or pay into the tax base that supports SSDI.

somatosensory nervous system: the receptors and processors that allow our senses to react to stimuli and comprehend things such as touch, temperature, body position, and pain.

spasm: a sudden tightening of muscles in an arm or leg. Spasms that occur at night are called nocturnal spasms.

spasticity: a chronic state of excessive muscle tone (too much tension in the muscles).

speech–language pathologist (SLP): the health care professional who focuses on speech and communication as well as swallowing problems. In MS, many SLPs also diagnose changes in thinking and memory and provide people with strategies to help manage them.

speech–language therapy: interventions provided by an SLP, including therapy for speech and swallowing problems and cognitive dysfunction.

sphincter muscle: any ringlike muscle surrounding a bodily opening that can open and close the opening. Sphincter muscles, which can be affected in MS, control the passage of urine and stool.

spinal cord: a cylindrical structure that runs through the center of the spinal column. It is full of nerve bundles that carry messages from your brain to the rest of your body and from your body up to your brain. Along with the brain and optic nerves, the spinal cord is part of the CNS.

stem cell: a cell that can develop into another type of cell.

structured exercise: planned exercises that are performed repeatedly over time with a specific goal, such as improved strength, endurance, balance, or flexibility.

support partner: any family member or friend who provides support and assistance on an ongoing basis to a person with MS. Also referred to as a care partner.

tertiary sexual problems: changes in sexual interest or activity due to attitudes or feelings that get in the way, including loss of self-esteem or self-confidence, an altered body image, or negative attitudes about illness or disability.

thoracic: refers to the area of the spine at the upper and middle part of the back, corresponding to the vertebrae T1–T12.

thyroid dysfunction: refers to any malfunction of the thyroid gland, including hypothyroidism (production of too little thyroid hormone) and hyperthyroidism (production of too much thyroid hormone).

tinnitus: the sound of ringing or buzzing in the ears that can occur in anyone and occasionally occurs in MS.

trans fats: fats that are produced by processing oils and adding hydrogen molecules to them. Like saturated fats, trans fats are thought to contribute to inflammation.

tremor: involuntary rhythmic movement of a given body part—usually an arm or leg, but it may also occur in the head and neck.

trigeminal nerve: the fifth cranial nerve, which provides sensation to the face.

trigeminal neuralgia: facial pain, sometimes quite intense, that travels along one or more of the three branches of the trigeminal nerve, which supplies sensation to the face.

trochlear nerves: the fourth pair of cranial nerves, which enable the eye to look downward or to look inward toward the nose.

urethra: a hollow tube that begins at the lower opening of the bladder and extends to the outside of the body. A woman's urethra carries urine out of the body; a man's urethra is used for both urination and ejaculation.

urinary catheter: a latex, polyurethane, or silicone tube that is inserted through the urethra into the bladder to allow urine to drain out of the body. A short, portable catheter can be used for intermittent self-catheterization; an indwelling catheter extends from inside the bladder to a collection bag outside the person's body.

urinary frequency: the urge to urinate many times during the day and night, even when the bladder is not full.

urinary tract infection (UTI): the presence of bacteria in the urinary tract that produces infection and symptoms such as burning with urination, urinating in small amounts, odor, fever, and chills. In people with MS, the symptoms may be different than those typically seen with a UTI and may include temporary worsening of MS symptoms such as mobility, spasticity, numbness, or other MS symptoms.

urinary urgency: the frequent urge to urinate immediately, even when the bladder is not full.

urodynamic testing: procedures conducted by a urologist or urogynecologist that examine how well parts of the urinary tract—bladder, sphincters, and urethra—are working to hold and empty urine.

urologist: a physician who specializes in male and female bladder function and male sexual function.

vascular comorbidities: common health conditions, which are known to hasten disease progression in people with MS, include high blood pressure, high cholesterol, heart disease, and diabetes.

vertigo: a symptom with many possible causes that generally results from an imbalance between the right and left vestibular symptom functions. An episode of vertigo can be momentary or last for an extended period.

vestibular rehabilitation (VRT): a specialized type of rehabilitation that can help improve balance. In VRT, exercises are used to help the vestibular system adapt in ways that increase gaze stability and posture stability, reduce symptoms of vertigo, and improve the ability to carry out activities of daily living.

vibratory sense: one of the discrimination senses that is tested during the neurologic exam. The examiner tests to determine whether the person can feel the vibrations of a tuning fork head against their skin.

virus: a submicroscopic infectious agent that replicates only inside living cells.

visual–spatial processing: a person's capacity to identify visual and spatial relationships. In MS, visuospatial problems might cause a person to get lost easily, feel disoriented, misjudge distances, or have difficulty with puzzles or objects that need to be assembled.

vitamin D: an essential nutrient that contributes to bone health, nerve conduction, mobility, and immune function. Despite being labeled a vitamin early in the 20th century, it is now considered a prohormone or hormone precursor.

walking poles: tools for walking or hiking that improve balance, posture, and endurance and are particularly helpful for walking uphill or downhill.

white matter: the deeper tissues within the brain and the outer tissues in the spinal cord that are covered with a protective coating of myelin, an insulating material.

working memory: a cognitive process with limited capacity that stores information temporarily. Examples include following multistep directions, remembering a thought as you wait for the other person to finish speaking, and remembering a phone number long enough to write it down.

worsening: occurs when a relapse does not completely resolve and leaves behind persistent symptoms.

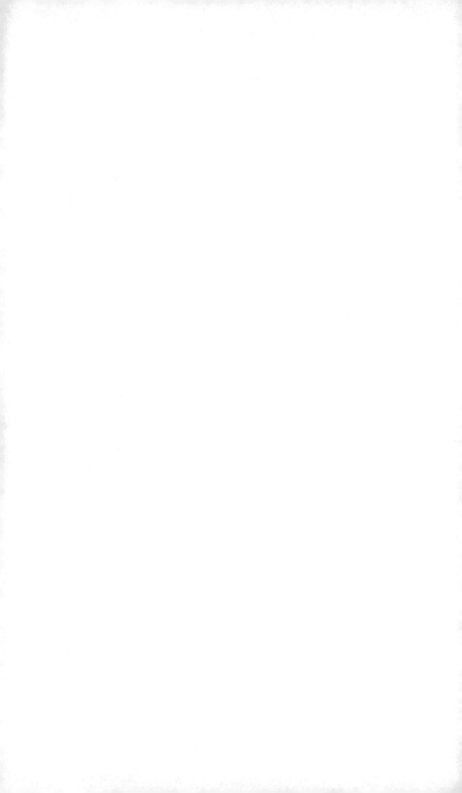

ABOUT *BRAIN & LIFE*® AND THE AMERICAN ACADEMY OF NEUROLOGY

The *Brain & Life*® family of products includes a magazine, website, podcast, and book series. A print subscription to *Brain & Life* (six issues a year) is available for free to anyone residing in the United States. Visit *BrainandLife.org* to subscribe and read stories on latest information on treatments, managing neurologic conditions, and advice for keeping your brain as healthy as possible.

Brain & Life is an official publication of the American Academy of Neurology (AAN), the world's largest community of neurologists and neuroscience professionals and a leading voice in brain health. The neurologists at the AAN are the minds behind *Brain & Life*. A neurologist is a doctor who specializes in the diagnosis, care, and treatment of brain, spinal cord, and nervous system diseases such as Alzheimer's disease, stroke, concussion, epilepsy, Parkinson's disease, multiple sclerosis, headache and migraine. Learn more about the AAN's commitment to brain health for all at *AAN.com*.

Kathleen Costello, CRNP, MSCN, is the Chief Operating Officer for Can Do Multiple Sclerosis, an organization dedicated to delivering health and wellness education for families living with MS. She is also adjunct faculty in the Division of Neuroimmunology and Neuroinfectious Diseases at the Johns Hopkins University School of Medicine in Baltimore, Maryland. She earned both her Bachelor of Science in Nursing and Master of Science degrees at the University of Maryland. She is a Board-certified Adult Nurse Practitioner and is also certified as an MS nurse. She specialized in MS care for more than 25 years in academic comprehensive care centers as a nurse and as a nurse practitioner at the University of Maryland and Johns Hopkins University Multiple Sclerosis Centers. She is a past president of the International Organization of Multiple Sclerosis Nurses and previously chaired the Multiple Sclerosis Specialist Certification Committee for the Consortium of Multiple Sclerosis Centers. She has worked with the Multiple Sclerosis International Federation on its successful efforts to add MS medications to the World Health Organization essential medicines list and has written and lectured extensively on MS and MS care.

Rosalind Kalb, PhD, CHC is Senior Programs Consultant for Can Do Multiple Sclerosis. She is a clinical psychologist, providing MS care and education for more than 40 years. After receiving her doctorate from Fordham University in New York, she provided mental health services and cognitive remediation at the Medical Rehabilitation Research and Training Center for Multiple Sclerosis at the Albert Einstein College of Medicine in New York City and later at the Multiple Sclerosis Comprehensive Care Center in White Plains, New York. She joined the National Multiple Sclerosis Society in 2000, creating on-line resources and educational materials for individuals and families living with MS and health care professionals until 2017.

Barbara S. Giesser, MD, FAAN, FANA, is Professor Emeritus of Clinical Neurology at the David Geffen UCLA School of Medicine and currently leads the MS program at Pacific Neuroscience Institute in Santa Monica, California. She is an internationally recognized clinician and award-winning educator who has specialized in the care of persons with MS for more than 40 years. She received her Bachelor of Science degree from the University of Miami, her Master of Science degree from the University of Texas School of Biomedical Sciences in Houston, and her Doctor of Medicine degree from the University of Texas Health Science Center at San Antonio. She completed her neurology residency at the Albert Einstein College of Medicine in New York City and did fellowship training in MS there at the Medical Rehabilitation Research and Training Center for Multiple Sclerosis. She was faculty at the Albert Einstein College of Medicine from 1983 until 1991 and was subsequently faculty at the University of Arizona Health Science Center before joining UCLA in 2002.

INDEX

For the benefit of digital users, indexed terms that span two pages (e.g., 52–53) may, on occasion, appear on only one of those pages

Tables, figures, and boxes are indicated by an italic *t*, *f*, and *b* following the page number.

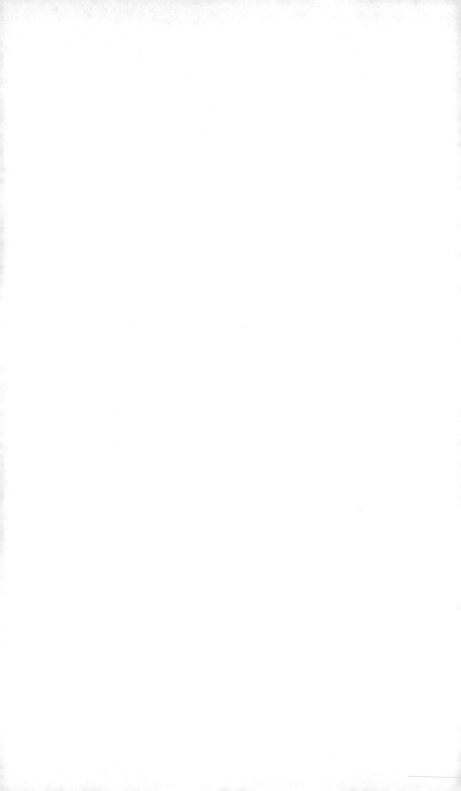